# FOOD ADDITIVES:
# THE TRUTH

## The True Story of Food Flavouring, Colouring and Preservatives, plus Much More

## What's In Your Food?

### *Food Conspiracy –Volume Three*

by Mark Plummer (B.Sc./PGCE)

www.viddapublishing.com

**This edition published by
VIDDA Publishing Ltd in 2018. www.viddapublishing.com
Copyright © VIDDA Publishing Ltd 2018**

Cover design by John Hodges.

# Table Of Contents

*For Helen*

*Without Her Love And Support*
*This Writing Would Not Be Here*

# An Opening Gambit – What to Expect and How to Read This Book

The writing presented here is an overview of a supremely complex issue. The text represents a tiny, almost non-existent scratch on a very large surface. This writing is not a novel. However, there are plenty of signposts so the reader can jump to different sections as they see fit. This book grew out of the research for my previous book "Food Conspiracy - What Happened To Our Bread? - The Chorleywood Bread Process". In a very real sense what you can see in front of you is a companion to that volume. Intensively manufactured or produced and large-scale food manufacturing all point toward the same subject and are used interchangeably. The use of the word construct refers to the whole global food processing business. I have looked at what is happening in the UK and the EU with a few mentions of the US and rest of the western world. Food regulations outside of the western world are much laxer than those which exist in the industrialised nations of this Earth. I absolutely dread to think what is occurring outside of the so called developed world, I really do. It is a safe bet that the less dangerous food additives banned here are pretty much available there. I have to clearly state that I am not an expert on this subject. I am what you might call a concerned citizen who is also a rational human being; I can see when things are not quite right. This writing is a result of a nose following exercise, that is, I am finding things out as I go along, then integrating new knowledge into that which already exists. Two years of research on this hugely complex issue has well and truly opened my eyes. It has also catalysed into meaningful action toward doing things differently. The writing here and on bread as well as GMO's has precipitated a real change in how my wonderful partner and I are going to live the rest of our lives. The hope is that the reader will consider doing the same. I didn't expect to discover food

1

processing to be a benign and fluffy operation. However, I did not expect the whole construct to be so woefully unregulated. I had no idea of how the industry itself is so totally unaccountable to the population that it is supposed to serve. I also did not expect the links between food processing, genetically modified food, the chemical industry and others to be as intertwined as they are. It is for these reasons that the tone of this writing is as uncompromising as it is hard-hitting. Most of the chapters provide an introductory section as to how the modern processed food industry, i.e. the construct, fits into the organisation of our affairs. Throughout this book, it will become ever more obvious that most modern additives can be used in different applications in different industries.

In a nutshell, this book will argue that the food industry has managed to gain control and concentrate so much power that genuinely avoiding processed food is impossible. The industry has this particular enterprise done up like a kipper. The first two chapters attempt to present the broad strokes as to why this is the case. Chapter two gives a snapshot as to what has been done to the food most of us have been eating over the decades leading up to 2017. Chapter two will also provide a picture of what may be just around the corner and the sort of machinations which could make it possible. Chapter three will impart how to avoid processed foods as best we can. Chapter four will give some real examples as to why you will want to. And chapter five will try to explain how things have gotten so messed up. Having said all of that, please do not be thinking this is an "anti-additives" or "anti-food processing book". It is not. There are plenty of techniques and substances that have been with us for many hundreds if not thousands of years and many of them are wholly beneficial. Also, there is nothing wrong in principle in upscaling a given method of food production. It is more the reasons why the processes are occurring in the first place that need questioning. Unless it is warranted the writing does not single out particular compounds or the class of chemical they belong to as dangerous. That has been done a thousand times or more and there is no need to re-invent a wheel that most of us can access via the internet. This book is more of a devastating critique of the industry itself and less an attack on particular additives, with perhaps chapters six and seven being the clearest cut examples of that position. I could have written a book on that subject alone and still had plenty left over for a second volume. As it is I have tried to present an overview of why it is that artificial sweeteners are not as benign as we have perhaps been led to believe. I certainly didn't know two years ago, what I now know about them. So if you are shocked, surprised and angered about what this chapter reveals then you are in good company. And that leads me to what will hopefully become another glaringly obvious point. By the time you have finished reading this volume, you will not want to eat any processed food at all. Want being the operative word! If anything said in this book resonates, then you are on the way to genuinely avoiding intensively produced food. The writing is an attempt to "tell it like it is" using as many disparate sources as possible, many of them from the industry and the science it sponsors. The reader, as usual, is absolutely encouraged to follow up on the references presented as they see fit. Any internet search will provide hundreds of examples of similar assertions and counter assertions concerning the kind of additives outlined in this text. The point to remember is that they are in the food you eat and the food you feed any children you may have.

Unless they are key decision makers I have to stress that I am not necessarily attacking people who work in the industry. It is the construct itself that deserves unrelenting flack. I mean to say most of us, if not all of us, have had to take employment with some thoroughly repugnant organisations to pay our way. So I am not throwing that stone in this particular glass house. How many of us have had jobs where we are paid wages by some pretty nasty organisations? I know I have and so once again, there is no intent to preach, berate or lecture. There is no abseiling or throat parachuting here! Aside from all other points, a future sustainable society is going to need the expertise of the food scientists employed. We are going to need them to be working with producers, growers, smallholders and soil scientists as well as others from just about every profession the reader can think of. In much the same way as we are going to need those employed in the nuclear industry to properly dismantle nuclear facilities, which in a sane world would not have been built at all; we are going to need "the experts" who are employed in "big agriculture". This position assumes that the person in question is not in some future dock for the crimes they have committed or more likely facilitated. The criminality I believe such people to be guilty of is highlighted throughout this book but particularly at the beginning of chapter two and throughout chapter three.

First and foremost this book is an overview. With reference to as many artificial substances, e numbers, additives, processing aids and otherwise approved chemicals, which I could cram in, the writing attempts to present the dire state of modern food production. So assuming you are still here, let's get going.......

# Chapter One: What Does Food Processing And Additive Use Really Mean?

Homo-sapiens are the only species of animal that routinely alter or process the food they eat. We are not the first. Food processing in its most basic form is an activity that stretches back into pre-history. An extinct species of bipedal (walking on two legs) hominid called Homo-erectus is believed to have discovered fire between one and two million years ago. I write discovered but what I really mean is this second species of bipedal hominid learned how to use fire. Wherever and however fire was first used, the ability would have spread rapidly across the range of the homo-erectus hominids. The previous bipedal species homo-habilis and the human-like organisms before them would have been aware of fire but according to the archaeological literature did not know how to employ it. If the evidence presents itself this supposition is subject to change. Irrespective of the whys, what's and wherefores, using fire was a pivotal development in our evolution. For our Pleistocene ancestors *"cooking"* food on *"the fire"* enabled more of the nutrients in the meat and/or fish to be metabolised and then assimilated when they were eaten as food. From a food perspective and since the use of fire bipedal hominids have been, altering, treating and adding substances to the collection of biological molecules we call food.[1] Using fire to cook these molecules into the meals we eat is the oldest form of food processing known to humanity. If you are looking for reasons as to why we enjoy a good Bar-B-Q this reality would be a good start. As a form of food processing using heat in the form of fire converts a *"raw"* food into a *"cooked"* form. From this start point we have, to put it bluntly, not looked back. Throughout our history, we have converted unprocessed plant and animal matter into the array of foods we call *"our diet"*. Processing food and later adding substances to it is a practice over a million years older than the Iron Age hill fort remains I can see from my study window. Fast forward two million years and here we are in the 21$^{st}$ century. In the modern age we "*process*" food for two basic reasons, one is preservation and the other is to make it more digestible. Or so the justifications from the manufacturers themselves inform us. If you listen to manufacturers, the techniques employed are for our benefit and are perfectly safe, provided that we follow their instructions. From that perspective, by altering and converting food from its "*natural*" or unprocessed state we are converting it into a more beneficial, i.e. more nutritious food. From this perspective, one would expect more of the good stuff to be in the processed form. If this line is to be believed we would also expect the nutrients to be more accessible to the human digestive system, meaning less of them are wasted. It is debatable as to whether this is the case and it will clearly depend on whom you ask. All animals including human beings ingest their food in a process called feeding. As soon as the food enters the animals mouth digestion begins. For some species of insects, digestion begins externally. For instance (minor spoiler alert), most of us have seen David Cronenberg's brilliant reworking of Kurt Neumann's 1958 Classic "*The Fly*". This absolutely must see classic piece of 1950's horror is based on a genuinely creepy short story of the same name by George Langelaan. What is perhaps a less well known fact is that the story was first published in the June 1957 issue of Playboy magazine. In the 1986 film version, Cronenberg's creation demonstrates his digestive prowess on camera by releasing digestive juices onto a plate of food and then sucking up the result through his proboscis, yum nice! So for a fly, digestion begins the instant the excreted juices make contact with the food. For mammals, digestion begins as soon as food enters the mouth and becomes subject to the attention of our teeth and any digestive enzymes in the saliva. So what is digestion? Digesting collections of biological molecules (i.e.

food) whether they are in a cooked or raw state is a highly complex biological process. For any animal, digestion has two basic objectives. First, it will be highly adapted to liberate as many nutrients as possible. Second, it will be equally adapted to provide as much chemical [2] energy as possible. Chemical energy is the form of energy bound up within food molecules themselves. Indeed all matter is held together by various types of chemical bonds. Every possible beneficial molecule and every joule of energy will be liberated from the food that is eaten. The rest is excreted. Both objectives are achieved by breaking large and insoluble (in water) biological molecules (i.e. proteins, carbohydrates and fats) into simpler and soluble molecules. The body can then assimilate the soluble molecules into the cells, tissues, organs and organ systems which make up the organism digesting the food. The digestive system of every organism on earth exists to fulfil these two essential functions. Why is digestion being explained? Well, because everything you eat is either excreted or becomes part of you and/or helps you function as you should. The chances are that just like myself you have eaten most of the substances mentioned in this book and plenty more besides. And you will have eaten them as part of your diet. Many of these substances are completely novel to human beings and the wider environment. Plenty of them are not subject to any real regulatory control. Some are added to your diet without your knowledge or consent. Some are more concerning than others and some are of no concern at all. For me this is not the point, I am more concerned with asking three deceptively simple questions:

- Why is substance X in our food in the first place?
- Where did X come from?
- What alternatives to substance X are there?

These three questions are the bedrock of this text. It is up to the reader to decide whether or not the questions or their implications are of any concern for them. I would think that most of us would want to know honest and clear answers to these questions. After all, the phrase *"you are what you eat"* means what it says. Every substance you eat or ingest comes into direct contact with you and your organ systems. With contact comes interaction and with interaction comes consequence. And that includes the nutrients in our food, traditional additives, plus every single synthetic or human made additive, which is in every mouthful of every meal that you have eaten until now and will eat until you draw your last breath.

A simple way to define a food additive is to frame it as any ingredient employed in the manufacture of processed food. A food additive is any substance, compound, chemical, powder, solid, liquid or solution that is added at any stage of the food manufacturing process. Processed foods contain the substances discussed in this book and the companion volume on modern bread making. These foods are packaged into boxes, cartons, bottles, cans, tubs, bags and other containers. As a general rule of thumb and good starting point, the longer the ingredient list, the more unpronounceable, unfamiliar or science sounding the substances are, the more likely the food is to have been processed. Here in the West, very little of what we eat is genuinely unprocessed. So, the next question has to be *"what is a processed food?"* In its loosest possible sense, a processed food is any food which has been converted from its *"natural"* state into an alternative form. So by definition, our Pleistocene ancestors were likely the first organisms on the Earth to process the food they ingested. For a food to be completely unprocessed it should not have been altered at all. For instance, meat and fish have been processed if they have been subject to any form of preservation, even salting, curing or smoking. If you look on the label of most processed meats you will also see water and various preservatives listed as added ingredients. Closer to home the soup I ate whilst reading this section of text was freshly made, frozen for a week, defrosted and then reheated in a microwave oven before finding its way back into my alimentary canal.

Surely a form of food processing and preservation, with deliciously impeccable results too! The distinction between *"processed"* and *"unprocessed"* is as easily blurred and ambiguous as the regulatory framework for the additives and processing techniques themselves. In this frame, we are not talking about *"traditional"*, *"artesian"* or *"historical"* methods of food processing, but modern and intensive methods of food production. Here the basic objectives are to:

- Improve and compliment the mechanisms through which the food itself is altered.
- Maintain the appearance, texture and consistency of the food being processed.
- Extend the transportation and shelf life of the finished product.
- Delay spoilage for as long as possible.
- Enhance the flavour, colour and taste of the finished product.
- Ensure that the *"true"* flavour, colour and taste of processed food are effectively concealed.

It is important to realise that food processing is not necessarily a bad idea or connected to some nefarious corporate intent. For instance, who in their right mind is going to suggest that cold pressing [3] nuts or olives to produce oils is undesirable? Or that adding spices and herbs to flavour food is somehow a bad idea? Exactly, no one! However, such techniques are not equivalent to adding preservatives to foods so that they can be transported for longer and have a longer shelf life. Nor are they equivalent to adding synthetic variants of nutrients that have been removed by the processing regime itself. Most vegetable oils, corn oils, soybean oils, or canola oils have been subject to bleaching (which removes colour from the oil), chemical extraction [4] and de-odourising. The mono-unsaturated oils which are converted to trans-fats are perhaps the most notorious (for the wrong reasons) of the processed oils. These oils and any foods which contain them most definitely fall under the definition *"processed"*. A further helpful but somewhat arbitrary marker between *"processed"* and *"un-processed"* might be whether you can pronounce the name of a given substance in the ingredients list. I have something of a science background, but I had to look up a hefty portion of the substances mentioned in this book. The reader could also read the label and ask whether you have heard of a listed ingredient or not. Even then the label does not often tell you very much. For instance, a brand of golden syrup from the supermarket simply states under the heading ingredients "golden syrup" and nothing else. Any quick internet search will inform that syrup is really a liquid form of sugar made by refining sugar. The sugar is likely derived from sugar cane. The syrup is made by separating sucrose into its constituent molecules fructose and glucose. A balance of sucrose and syrup is then established depending on the type of syrup in question. The label tells us nothing about where the sugar cane comes from. I cannot tell if it comes from genetically engineered sugar cane or not. I have no idea which preservatives are used and why they are present. The particular container I am looking at right now has solidified so I'm assuming it has been in the larder for a good few months. It shows no sign of spoilage. So I'm guessing it must have some sort of preservative added to it. The point is I don't know and I have no real way of finding out. Any ingredients listed and plenty that are not are going to find their way into your digestive system. From there, they are going to be distributed throughout your body by one mechanism or another. Generally speaking, most of the substances which compose intensively produced food would be somewhat out of place in the superb and well-thumbed farmhouse cookbook which has pride of place in our tiny kitchen. Processed foods generally contain ingredients with long unpronounceable names. The writing is tiny and the words and/or numbers tell you nothing about what the additive ingredient does or why it is present. To find out the only recourse is to research the compound and the processes and/or industries which use it. This is no easy task, as anyone (including yours truly) who has tried will attest. A recurring question with food processing is to politely inquire, *"If the manufacturers of the food we eat are so concerned with safety, quality, health and sustainability, why is there such an opaque shroud of secrecy around their practices"*? One of those practices is outlined in the next section.

## Nutrification is Fortifying and Enriching

Fortification and enrichment are mentioned again in chapter four. The earliest example of supplementation of food I came across occurred approximately 2500 years ago, on a Tuesday at about three 'o' clock in the afternoon. A Persian physician called Melanpus came up with an ingenious idea. He apparently suggested adding iron filings to the wine given to soldiers before they went into the organised slaughter and carnage of ancient world battlefields. The iron was believed to increase aggression and therefore the proclivity to kill. Ingenious you see, and for today I wonder what pills, potions and powders are given to armed forces personnel today. Later, in early 19$^{th}$ century France, iodine was first added to common salt to prevent the formation of goitres. We can legitimately ask what it was about the French diet that meant such additions were necessary. Clearly, identical questions can be asked about the food we all eat in the 21$^{st}$ century world. It was after the First World War that supplementation by enrichment and fortification really took off. Since then the industry has never looked back. Nutrification has been taken to a new and thoroughly undesirable level. The food processing under discussion in this book almost always degrades its nutritional qualities. For instance, the *"Food Conspiracy"* book outlines how iron and B vitamins are added to wheat flour after it has been milled and separated. Similarly, vitamins A and D are added to margarine so that it has some similarity to unprocessed butter, (see butter buds in chapter 2). These are but two examples of enrichment, where a substance is added to replace those lost during the processing itself. Fortification is concerned with adding substances which are not present in the unprocessed form of the food. For instance, calcium is added to some fruit juices which is supposed to boost the skeletal system of people who do not eat dairy products. Further examples are mentioned in chapter four. As far as the manufacturers are concerned enrichment and fortification are important sources of nutrients that we otherwise would not have access to. Various statutes concerning permissible levels of added nutrients are in place. The levels themselves are based on the results of scientific experiment. Through a prism of public health, enrichment and fortification in specific examples absolutely have their place. Yet, such a statement does not address why a given deficiency is occurring in the first place. The same question can be asked of those who support GMO's for nutritional reasons. Similarly, if the reason for *"nutrification"* (enrichment and fortification) is due to the processing regimes themselves then clearly questions are going to be asked. If nutrification is carried out to increase the nutritional qualities of *"unhealthy"* food, then further questions concerning the quality of the food have to be asked. In this setting, the questions have to focus on what is being made and why. We have to ask the three basic questions posed above. For example, there is no nutritional point in adding synthetic forms of nutrients to a high salt, processed or junk food. Such activity clearly misses the point entirely. If the processing itself is causing the nutrient depletion then surely the answer has to be to stop the processing. However, as chapters two and three clearly impart this is not going to happen any time soon.

As we approach the end of 2017, in excess of thousands of individual human made or synthesized chemicals exist in the human food chain, (see chapter four). They are added under the respective banners of *"enrichment"* and *"fortification"* and absolutely all of them have a stated purpose. Whether the purpose is a good idea or not is a point open to interpretation and perception. Other substances are added under the heading *"preservative"*, or employed as *"processing aids"*. Often the industry and food manufacturers do not have to inform as to the presence of a given substance. And so it goes on and on.....These realities do not include the plethora of chemicals, growth hormones and antibiotics used in the intensive rearing of fish, livestock and any animal products thereof. Pretty much every food processing regime in existence degrades the nutritional quality of the food it alters. If they didn't I would not have written this book or its companion volume. Symptoms of this loss in quality are changes in the texture, appearance, flavour and taste of the finished product. If most of us were to see what part processed food really looks like, I'm sure we would not be impressed. I know I wasn't and what I have found out during the course of putting this book together has, to put it mildly, left me somewhat upset. The reader is encouraged to follow up on the references themselves and not just take my word for it. To put it politely un-altered *"raw processed"* food is visually unappealing, is not palatable and would elicit the *"yuck factor"* response (see chapter two) in any rational person. One particular lie concerning the quality of food in the Western diet concerns what we are told is the most important meal of any day. Breakfast cereals generally express their nutritional qualities in such a way that you cannot miss them. What the producers don't tell you is that the raw form of the cereal, whether it be corn or grains is mixed with water and mulched into an off-white coloured slurry. The slurry is then fed into a processing machine called an extruder. The machine functions by forcing the slurry through a variety of different tiny holes, depending on the cereal being made. The slurry is fed through the shapes at high pressure and temperature and the result is individual shapes, flakes or shredded forms of the original food. The extruded form is then sprayed with various preservatives, drying agents (which provide the crunch) and a molecule thin layer of oil to prevent oxidation (staling) once the cereal is opened. The extruded cereal has virtually no nutritional content. Once subject to these processes the original vitamins and minerals are utterly destroyed. For instance, the amino acid lysine is particularly vulnerable to the stresses of extrusion. Many of the original and beneficial oils and fatty acids are annihilated. The slurry itself looks (and probably tastes) disgusting and is thoroughly unappealing. All the nutrification and adding of colourants happens at the end of the processing. I don't really eat breakfast cereals but if I did they would most certainly feature in chapter three.

Humanity is now in a despiculous (fusion of despicable and ridiculous) position whereby the nutrification and processing of food is now the norm. Fresh, wholesome, healthy and nutritious food is the exception and can with some justification be seen as some sort of status symbol for those that can afford to eat it. This point is hammered home in chapter three. Nutrification has not eliminated vitamin and mineral deficiencies; it has replaced one set of problems for another. Altering food under the auspices of the Western diet has caused a whole new set of health and nutritional problems. It seems sensible to ask some questions to back up this assertion:

- Why is it necessary to fortify and enrich processed foods in the first place?
- What is it about the food we eat in the first place that makes nutrification necessary?
- Why is that so many of these deficiencies tend to hurt particular sections (i.e. the poor) of society?
- Why is it that in populations filled with supposedly well-nourished and affluent people, there are so many unnecessary health issues in the first place?
- How can the right dose of a given *"fortificant"* be set for a given population?
- How can a given dose be set so that it is effective but not toxic?
- How can the proponents of fortification be so sure that

other unforeseen toxic or unhealthy impacts do not present themselves?

Likely, most of the existing nutritional problems would not be anything like as prevalent if processing and adulteration were kept to an absolutely necessary minimum. Yet, it isn't and now we are over halfway through the second decade of the 21ˢᵗ century. The consequences of two centuries of big business controlled food processing and adulteration are clear to those who are looking. The *"medicine on your plate"* series makes absolutely clear that a well-balanced diet will help in the prevention of many diseases. The self-inflicted global obesity epidemic perhaps is the most well-known example. However, we are also looking at lower growth rates for children and young people and increasing rates of arthritis and atherosclerosis in older populations. We are also looking at deficiencies in folic acid and folate and in trace minerals. Undoubtedly the Western diet is playing its part in the steady increase in global cancer rates and reductions in life expectancy too. No amount of fortification can ever take the place of a genuinely balanced diet. A diet which in a sane world would be composed of affordable and accessible, fresh, nutritious and wholesome food. To state that *"fortification"* can substitute for *"fresh"* is to imply that substances added to food for *"health"* reasons are somehow more effective than those which already exist. Clearly, such a position is as nonsensical as it is oxymoronic, isn't it? However, it seems the food industry and its apologist supporters disagree! These issues are complex and there is no single cause, one cannot lay *"the ills of the world"* solely at the doors of intensive food production. However, we can say with absolute clarity that it is a contributory factor to the current disgusting and inhumane state of the health of people and planet.

## Natural or Artificial? You Tell Me!

For the purpose of this writing, a food is processed if it contains (or has employed the use of any additive) during its manufacture. Therefore an additive is any substance necessary for the manufacture of processed food. A processed food does not solely mean ready, microwave or take away meals but refers to ANY food that has been altered for whatever reason from its *"natural"* state. The word *"natural"* in the world of food production is highly subjective and almost impossible to define explicitly. A food cannot be seen as natural if it contains substances which are not found in the natural world, even if the chemical in question is a direct copy of the natural form. A food cannot be considered natural if it has been subject to enrichment (see below) or has been subject to vagaries of genetic modification. The definition becomes even murkier when we start looking at cross and selective breeding, extraction of natural chemicals and the role of genetically engineered crops and animals in modern agriculture. Many of the staple food crops and animals reared or farmed by intensive methods would be completely unrecognisable as *"natural"* to even our grandparents. Within the definition of nutrification, there are plenty of examples of additives which have been with us for hundreds of years or longer (see chapter four) which are not in any way problematic. Conversely and most definitely, natural does not always mean good or harmless.

If a substance has been added or employed to produce a food, by definition, the food has been processed or adulterated. It can be argued that potatoes from the supermarket are processed because they have been washed and transported in a plastic bag. Following on, chapter three will make clear that avoiding processed food is for all intents and purposes impossible. Most of us are eating far more of it than we realise. As for the processing itself, the individual techniques employed by the food industry come under headings including:

- Freezing and refrigeration
- Preserving
- Smoking

- Freeze drying
- Vacuum Packing
- Salting
- Sweetening
- Pickling
- Fermentation
- Canning
- Dehydrating
- Irradiation
- Pasteurisation
- Nutrification

It is obvious that such techniques have completely and negatively skewed our relationship with the food we eat. Clearly, some are more controversial than others plus the techniques are not necessarily bad practices in themselves, yet, this misses the point entirely. Given a straight and financially unencumbered choice, I would rather eat unprocessed, fresh, locally sourced and/or seasonal foods where my hard earned went into the coffers of the nearest grower or producer and not to a construct I despise. Notions of additives, e-numbers and preservatives tap into this line of reasoning. If the global food distribution system were organised differently and had objectives which extended beyond profit we would not need to have discussions about processed foods because most of them would not exist. Clearly, not all additives or food processing techniques are in themselves detrimental to human health, animal welfare and sustainability in food production and distribution. Science and history teach us that very often the opposite holds true. It is obvious that any food left for long enough will eventually spoil. In principle, there is absolutely nothing wrong with preserving food for as long as possible. For example, chapter five outlines how meat and meat products have been preserved both today and in the past. Leaving aside the ethical and environmental issues concerning eating meat, it is difficult to argue against such preservation techniques.

However, pickling surplus vegetables in vinegar and storing them in a sealed glass container is not the same as adding synthetic chemicals to a given food so that it can sit on a supermarket shelf for several weeks and be labelled as fresh and wholesome. Closer to home I am able to pick plenty of fruit straight from the plants for the kitchen and for the making of wine. This fruit is in the freezer and has been for several months now. It will be time to start picking again by the time the freezer is empty. I have a bigger gripe in that the appliance itself is powered by the combustion of fossil fuels, likely with a healthy portion of nuclear power too.

## Cross Links Aplenty

From a food perspective, the 21st century is characterised by the prolific use of additives, processing aids and the techniques which facilitate their use. If one takes a look at how any processed food is made it becomes clear that the additives and processing regimes cannot exist without each other. The substitution of *"natural"* or *"whole"* substances for synthetic variants and other substances is routine. Individual examples are mentioned throughout this book. Modern processed food is filled with a bewildering array of substances. Most of them really do not have any business being in any food, or for that matter anywhere else. Intensively made food is laden with artificial dyes, colourants, emulsifiers, sweeteners, artificial flavours and enhancers. And that is merely the ingredients the industry is obliged to tell you about. Many of these substances are manufactured by the chemical and petro-chemical industries. The products of refining crude oil or the derivatives of coal are present in mass produced processed food. For instance:

- Propyl Gallate (E 310) [5]: An ester compound formed when proponal (an alcohol) chemically bonds to gallic acid. It is an anti-oxidant which prevents lipids (fats and oils) from reacting with oxygen. When lipids react with oxygen they become oxidised. They are said to have turned rancid. Esters form when any alcohol is chemically bonded to an organic (carbon based, fatty or carboxylic) acid.

Triglycerides are esters because three fatty acids bond with a molecule of glycerol (another alcohol). Esters are hugely important molecules and are discussed in the Chorleywood Bread Process book.

- Butylated Hydroxy-anisole (BHA E 320) [6] see chapter two: An example of what chemists refer to as an aromatic compound.[7] These compounds contain a structure called a benzene ring which gives the compound its unique *"aromatic"* characteristics. This particular aromatic compound prevents fats from turning rancid, i.e. it slows the oxidation [8] of fats.

- Tertiary Butyl-hydroquinone (TBH E 319 [9]): Another aromatic compound which is also a phenol. It is exceptionally efficient in preventing the oxidation of unsaturated oils and animal fats. Phenols [10] are formed when a hydroxyl (OH) functional group [11] bonds directly to a carbon atom on a benzene ring. Phenols are mentioned in the medicine on your plate series of books.

Along with the chemicals added to fertilisers, we are almost certainly eating derivatives of both the fractional distillation [12] and subsequent catalytic cracking [13] of crude oil components. Clear and present links exist between intensive agriculture, the oil business, the wider chemical industry and the food manufacturers. Consequently, they end up in the food you eat. Such substances are but one fraction of the substances added to processed food. In this writers view they cannot be considered *"natural"* or *"wholesome"* in any manner whatsoever. They should not be there; they should be in the place the fossil fuel they came from, in the ground.

The processed food industry invests a huge amount of time, money and expertise into developing artificial flavours and colourants. Globally, the industry defends its interests by using language and legal statute that would put the linguists behind doublespeak to shame. The flavourings and colourants are needed to mask the taste consequences of producing the commodity we know as processed food. Further demonstrating the links between the wider chemical industry and the processed food sector which part composes it, many identical substances are listed in different processed foods. I don't need to put any examples in here you will find plenty in your food cupboard, so please do go and have a look. See, there you go! Many of these substances have different utility in different industries. For instance, anti-ageing creams contain *"phyto-sterols"* [14] and *"polyunsaturated fatty acids"*, derived from soy beans. The phyto-sterols are found in most plants and (amongst other roles) inhibit the absorption of cholesterol and low density lipo-proteins [15] (LDLP) from the human gut into the general circulation. In moderation, polyunsaturated fats have demonstrable benefits for human cardiovascular health. The point is that the same substances are used by two different industries for completely different purposes. For this example, it is the cosmetics industry and the food processing industry. How about a second example? Oh, go on then, while we are here! An enzyme called Co-enzyme Q10 [16] has a vital role to play in the corpus of biochemical reactions which we collectively call *"aerobic respiration"*. It is one of the many synthetic chemicals manufactured by means of genetically engineered microbes [17] and/or by various fermentation techniques. Aside from cosmetics it is also used extensively in pharmaceuticals and is a favourite of the food supplement and other industries. Such substances are representative of "big business" [18] and its objectives. Any beauty product which states *"from soya"* is almost certain to contain GMO's or their derivatives. Biotechnology in the form of GMO's is well and truly entrenched in both industries. As with many aspects of our lives, it is the construct (big pharma / the food industry) which is the problem and not necessarily the substance itself. I don't believe that people who are employed in such industries are necessarily the problem either. After all, who can honestly say they have never had a job with one of *"the man's"* employers to pay the rent,

I know I have. I'm willing to bet most if not all of you out there have too.

Not bothered, phased or convinced by any of this?

How about another example?

The vast majority of salmon available in supermarkets today comes from aquaculture (fish farms). Leaving aside the choice to eat seafood in the first place, price constraints mean that avoiding farmed or canned fish is a false choice for most people. If you don't have the readies you are not going to buy fish procured through genuinely sustainable sources. Where I live organic, freshly caught and wild salmon costs over three times the farmed variety. There is a wholefood supermarket about two miles from where I live. If I wish to buy one tuna steak which is certified organic, pole and line caught I am looking at wallet eating amounts of cash. A responsibly farmed alternative is available, but it still costs considerably more than standard supermarket fare. I don't blame the food outlet at all; I blame the food system and the wider construct of which it is a part. So, what is the problem here? Most important, salmon and any other fish reared by intensive aquaculture are not living in their natural environment. Clearly, the same is going to apply to the GM salmon which is becoming increasingly available. The fish do not have access to their natural food sources. In the wild salmon eat crustaceans, which contain a substance called astaxanthin.[19] The compound is one of the most potent anti-oxidants in the natural world and is also a carotenoid. [20] It gives salmon flesh and tissues its characteristic pink colour. It is designated as E 161 along with eight individual [21] astaxanthin compounds. In a farmed environment astaxanthin is one of the many chemicals added to the animals' feed pellets. The substance gained approval [22] for use in fish farming and as a supplement across the EU in 2008. Personally, though, I'm not sure about the wisdom of partaking of it on a daily basis. Synthetic astaxanthin [23] is one of the thousands of artificial compounds that the European Food Safety Authority (EFSA – whose web page is listed below) maintains is safe for human consumption. These experiments are conducted in isolation from the thousands of other compounds which the same agency marks as safe. The recurrent and essential point (which is repeatedly raised throughout this writing) and fundamental question has been missed. Which is to ask, *"why are such compounds put into the food most of us eat"?* We also need to ask *"why is so much salmon farmed"?* The second question has to be answered in terms of what is being done to biodiversity in the oceans of the planet we all live on, which is not the subject of this book. The first question can be answered with reference to how industrial food processing works, i.e. with reference to the titular question of this chapter. Up until recently coal tar [24] was an important precursor compound for a whole range of food additives. Raw coal tar is a black liquid produced when coal is converted to coke and smokeless fuels. As with methane gas from oil wells, coal tar was at first seen as a waste product from coal mining. The tar contains thousands of individual compounds of which some are known carcinogens. The World Health Organisation (WHO) states that any solution containing 5% coal tar marks the boundary between carcinogenic and non-carcinogenic. In the mid-19th century, coal tar was elevated from waste product to treasure trove of useful compounds. The nascent pharmaceutical industry began using coal tar as a source of substances to profit from. Any chemist who had the ability to create new beneficial substances stood to make their fortune. Again, there is nothing wrong with exploiting naturally occurring beneficial substances. There is everything wrong with a construct which puts profit above all other considerations. The same oil based and synthetic variants are today used across the smorgasbord of industrial activities which keep the current economic system functioning. Returning to salmon and underlining the point about how opaque industrial food processing really is, it is difficult to say categorically that compounds derived from coal tar are no longer used by the food industry. Some sources say they are and some say they are not. It is absolutely true to state that the astaxanthin used in intensive aquaculture is derived from crude oil refining, i.e. the petrochemical industry. The astaxanthin gives the fish a false pink colour, without it the salmon flesh would be a pale white colour. It is added to the salmon feed for the same reason that the colourants and other substances are added to extruded breakfast cereals. The synthetic astaxanthin is used to hide the real colour of the farmed fish. Remember, this is just one facet of one part of a giant global construct. I wonder what else has been done to mask the real appearance of farmed salmon in particular and farmed fish in general.

A visit to any supermarket provides a visual demonstration of the illusion of food choice. We are all bombarded with it on a daily basis or every time you walk along any high street in Britain. This false choice is composed of the foods which collectively make up the justifiably eviscerated western diet. A diet characterised by excessive amounts of salt, refined sugars and saturated fats is not over a lifetime going to be free from issues. This diet is also a byword for words including:

- Additive
- Emulsifier
- Artificial Colour
- Artificial Flavour
- Artificial sweetener
- Enhancer
- Enzymes
- Preservatives (shelf life extenders)
- E number
- Processing aids

A glance at the label of any individual processed food reveals the blatantly obvious. Each of these headings represents a confusing assemblage of substances, which most of us have never heard of. Some of these compounds are entirely natural substances, except increasingly they are not! Again, it is important to state that synthetic does not always mean toxic; it is more a question of the use of additives per se. For instance, with vitamin E or the tocopherols (E 306-309 [25]) the natural variant is called d-alpha tocopherol and the synthetic variant is called dl-alpha tocopherol. Along with vitamin C [26] (E 300 whose manufacture is mentioned in the *"Food Conspiracy"* book) the tocopherols are very effective anti-oxidants. They are useful preservatives because they prevent the onset of rancidity in animal fats. Naturally, vitamin E is found in nuts, fish, leafy green vegetables and vegetable oils. Most ready meals are loaded to the max with anti-oxidants. Skin care beauty products contain synthetic copies of tocopherol compounds. In this example, I am not aware of any evidence that the synthetic form is toxic (under normal circumstances) to human beings. Again this assertion misses the point entirely, the reader should be aware of this every time food issues crop up in their life. The synthetic form is significantly less effective as an anti-oxidant than the natural form. So, Mexican waves everybody, people prefer the natural form. Another example could be the natural sleep aid Melatonin. [27] The natural form of this sleep regulating hormone is derived from the pineal gland of mammals. In this form, it can contain viral material which can become pathogenic in some people. Accordingly, the synthetic copy is exactly that, an exact chemical duplicate. However, the risk of pathenogenesis (illness) is removed because the copy contains no viral material. If you are of a vegan or vegetarian persuasion the reasons for taking the synthetic version ought to be obvious. Clearly, if you are struggling to sleep, then finding out why has to be given priority. The list of synthetic examples is truly endless and constantly expanding. The lecithin used by the food industry to create emulsions is just one conduit for refined chemicals to enter the human food chain. Loosely defined an emulsifier is any substance that prevents two liquids from separating. The liquids are suspended and in direct contact with each other in a solution. Lecithin carries the number E 322 [28] and the commercial forms are mainly derived from egg yolks or soy beans. The seeds which grew into the beans are almost certain to have been genetically modified. This deliberate muddying of the waters is one reason why GMO's are present in the food we eat. Sadly, as discussed in the Introducing GMO's book, there are plenty more. The sleight of hand means that GM soy beans themselves are not used directly in food manufacture, but chemicals derived from them can be, in this case, the lecithins. This will not be the only example. Exactly the same happens with animal livestock feed and fish meal. Naturally, lecithin is found in the cell walls of most plants. Lecithin is not a single substance. In modern food processing, the lecithins are a family of slightly different compounds. For instance, partially hydrolysed Lecithin is denoted as E 322 (ii). Their basic purpose is to stop different fats and oils separating. The lecithin used in the food industry is certain to have been highly processed, refined and purified. Hydrolysis means that protein molecules have been partially broken down into their constituent amino acids. The degree of breakdown (hydrolysis) of the protein (in this case the lecithin) is generally measured against the stability [29] of the emulsion. Clearly, different foods are going to require differing degrees of hydrolysis. The manufacturers are under no obligation to declare the source of lecithin or production techniques involved in its manufacture. This reality applies to the whole industry and cellulose is another supremely relevant example.

## Cellulose

Cellulose is merely one instance of an additive derived from ostensibly natural sources. Cellulose is an exceptionally long unbranched chain of glucose molecules which are chemically bonded to each other; it is a long chain carbohydrate. The structure which makes the bonding possible is called a glycosidic bond. Cellulose is the main component of the cell wall in all plant cells, most algae and some fungi. One of its many functions is to provide rigidity to the cell. The rigidity provides structure and cohesion for the whole organism. For instance, when plant cells take on water they expand. The expansion pushes the cell against its cell wall (i.e. the cellulose) and the cell can expand no further. This is known as turgidity which enables the plant to stand firm. If the plant loses too much water, its turgidity begins to diminish and the plant begins to wilt. Without cellulose, turgidity would be impossible. Well thanks for the science lesson Mark, but what does this have to do with food? Well, if you ever see the phrase *"processed wood pulp"* on the ingredients list, the cellulose has almost certainly come from trees. Cellulose is a well recognised and beneficial source of dietary fibre. Whether or not it should be derived from wood pulp is another matter. Depending on how it is to be used the cellulose can be kept in fibrous form or converted to powder. The wood is cooked in various chemicals to separate the cellulose from the rest of the wood components. Pure cellulose is denoted by the number E 460. [30] Once separated cellulose has a multitude of uses in food and textile manufacturing. The cellulose used to manufacture garments and carpets is the same molecule present in the food we eat. The same physical properties which allow plants and trees to stand also provide structure and water retention properties for pies, pastries and cake mixes. Pulped cellulose is used to stabilise and thicken intensively made food as well as the sauces and other liquids they contain. These various forms of cellulose are used in cheeses, salad dressings, condiments, syrups, condiments, jams, muffins and crumpets. It is entirely possible that the golden syrup mentioned above contains cellulose, but I have no easy and reliable method for finding out. The fast food industry employs powdered [31] cellulose as a means to bulk out its various food products.[32] The practice increases profits because you are buying as much cellulose that the industry can get away with selling to you.

Substituting ingredients in any food for cellulose represents another gravy train for the processed food industry. Using cellulose reduces fast food processing costs by any quantity up to 30 percent.[33] Replacing as many ingredients as possible for powdered cellulose is going to be a supremely attractive proposition to an industry where the bottom line is everything. Cellulose is non-poisonous and edible but is not readily digested in the human alimentary canal. In situ, that is in the plant it came from, cellulose has clear benefits for the digestive process, but it has no nutritional value whatsoever. In powdered or chopped form it acts as a bulking and stabilising agent for hundreds of individual foods. As far as I am aware there is no restriction on the quantity or sourcing of the cellulose (or its derivatives), used in processed foods. The regulatory authorities have no real interest in moderating, restricting or halting the use of wood derived cellulose. The number E 460 delimits only a precursor molecule, i.e. the cellulose itself. This e number does not refer to any individual compounds which are made from it. There are an additional 9 substances labelled from E 461 to E469 [34] inclusive. The compounds which contain cellulose belong to an entire class of chemicals which number at least several dozen in total. This larger family of molecules are known as hydro colloids,[35] are also discussed in the *"Food Conspiracy"* book. They have several roles, one of them is to function as thickening or gelling agents and this occurs because they are able to absorb and retain water.

The use of cellulose and other substances outside of food production is not supposed to upset us. For instance, one manufacturer of hydrocolloids called cyber colloids (see website below) and those who adhere to notions of *"modernist cooking"* or *"precision agriculture"* (i.e. GM crops) wear and promote the multiple uses of chemicals in food as a badge of virtue.[36] The two terms in italics tell you all you need to know about the future the processed food industry has in store if it is allowed to continue.

I'm sure if you consider yourself to be a savvy consumer with your finger on the pulse with all the hipstering that entails, you'll find such developments thoroughly absorbing. This potential future is outlined in chapter two. Personally, I choose to reject it wholesale as best I can, whenever I can. The hydrocolloids are also of great importance to the cosmetics industry. As they retain water they are ubiquitous in skin treatment products. The food industry can and does frame using cellulose and its derivatives (through the science it funds) as entirely "natural". [37] From this perspective, cellulose is not particularly problematic and at face value why should it be? However, the devil, as they say, is in the detail and the two obvious questions mentioned above again present themselves. First, *"what is cellulose from wood pulp doing in our food in the first place"?* Second, *"From what wood source does the cellulose come from?* We have already answered question one. It is all about the green, end of story! All other points are a distracting matrix of smoke and mirrors. As for question two, well, you tell me? Cellulose is often further processed and altered to suit a particular application, it can also be:

- E 426 Soybean hemicellulose (almost certainly from a GM soya source).
- E 460 Cellulose.
- E 461 Methyl Cellulose.
- E 462 Ethyl Cellulose.
- E 464 Hydroxypropyl Methyl Cellulose.
- E 465 Ethyl Methyl Cellulose.
- E 466 Sodium Carboxy Methyl Cellulose (Cellulose Gum).
- E 468 Cross Linked Sodium Carboxy Methyl Cellulose (Cross linked Cellulose Gum).
- E 469 Enzymatically Hydrolysed Carboxy Methyl Cellulose (Enzymatically Hydrolysed Cellulose Gum).
  - E 1525 Hydroxyethyl Cellulose.

So the next time somebody in your life refers to cellulose as *"natural"* ask them to explain how the above list of substances came to be in our food and what they are used for. Pulped cellulose and its various derivatives are used to replace fats and bulking agents whilst increasing the fibre content. None of these substances provide any nutritional value to the food we eat. They cannot by definition be considered a food. They can by definition be referred to as some of the several thousand substances known as food additives.

## Eggs

The processed food industry is a human construct. It exists solely to make a profit, it has no other purpose. This book ought to make this underlying point a glaring and deeply uncomfortable reality. The construct itself is really just one of the many oligarchs which compete ruthlessly with each other for the cash you possess. Most of what you see on the supermarket shelves are different brand names owned by the same very few, but seriously large transnational corporations. As chapter two demonstrates they will strive for ever more technically brilliant methods to substitute *"expensive"* for *"inexpensive"* ingredients and combinations thereof. As chapter six on aspartame demonstrates there is no trick or depth too low to stoop in the pursuit of relieving you of your money. The industry is not shy about covering its rather nefarious tricks in the economic, political and scientific trade within which it operates. The intensive food industry and the *"big agriculture"* construct it is part of have abdicated their responsibility to the people they are supposed to feed. They have managed to project their collective culpability with some success on to the people they have so successfully deceived too. The construct and its representatives maintain they are only meeting a demand for the foods we want to buy. Some additives and processing techniques are clearly beneficial and necessary but many more are not. For instance, the Campden tablets which sterilise my winemaking equipment and the wine itself provide Sulphur dioxide [38] ($SO_2$), E 220 [39]. Once liberated the gas readily dissolves in water forming a very weak solution of sulphuric acid. Along with all the other acids produced during fermentation, the wine becomes far too acidic for mould and bacteria to grow. It also functions as a very powerful anti-oxidant and has been used in this capacity by the beverages industry for many decades. This particular beneficial use of a natural substance has been with us since the time of Melanpus. Conversely, the unnecessary additives exist only to generate profit for the industry. In this context the pertinent question is to ask:

- Who decides what is necessary whose judgement do we trust and why do we trust it?
- Do we trust the current construct or do we trust those who are working toward genuine food security and sustainability?
- When it comes to discussions on the scientific basis or the toxicology of substances do we trust communications from the industry and/or *"the establishment"*?
- Do we trust scientific research and communications concerning it from other agencies?

Leaving aside that for most of us choosing the best quality food is a false choice, (see chapter three). For the above and any other questions the reader may have, it depends on your own level of acceptance of what you are prepared to put up with. It also depends on what you are prepared to feed any children you may have, which brings us to the humble but ubiquitous standard chicken egg. A good place to start with this particular staple food is the catastrophe (which far too many people here in the UK still see as a celebration) known as the Second World War.

The second global conflict made food rationing an absolute necessity for the survival of Britain and its people. Make no mistake about it, only the *"dig for victory campaign"* prevented nationwide hunger if not flat out Yemeni style starvation and disease. The cause of that particular genocidal crime against humanity is the regime in Saudi Arabia, its principal backers the

US government and its confused imperialist poodle also known as UK plc. Anyway back to more avoidable genocide and organised mass murder, a people cull if you will. Even before the second avoidable global conflict, powdered eggs were supplied as a cheaper substitute for the real thing. However, *"during the war"* dried and powdered eggs became a substitute for real eggs. Today, powdered eggs are supplied with added sugar, salt and essential nutrients. Be assured, these substances are added in an attempt to replace the forms which were present in the unprocessed egg. The replacement nutrients are likely to be synthetic copies of real vitamins or they will have been extracted from other foods. Equally, they could be a combination of both. Anybody who has cooked with eggs knows that they can be separated into the yolk and albumen. I have even used the yolk to froth up my favourite cocktail, the most amazing amaretto sour. The albumen has then found use as a binding material in egg white omelettes. The use of an egg in such ways is a far cry from what happens to them when they are processed. In the world of intensive food processing, the albumen is treated with gels and emulsifiers which enables more rapid whipping of the white. Eggs which find their way into industrial food production can be:

- Separated
- Pasteurised
- Frozen
- Dehydrated
- Crystallised
- Chilled
- Suspended
- Preserved

The basic need for these techniques is to use the eggs in other foods or to extend the shelf and therefore transportation life of the eggs themselves. I grew up in Brussels and in very short order developed a taste for frites. And that means I developed a taste for

31

dipping them in sauces, including my favourite dipping sauce of all time, andalouse. As most of us know egg yolk is a key component of mayonnaise. Until we started making our own I had no idea how much oil is in the average serving of this most wonderful condiment. We still buy it regularly and use it to make andalouse sauce and another personal favourite, garlic mayonnaise. However, we have stopped buying the low-fat variety. Which may sound counter intuitive, but the following ingredients list should explain why. In the mass production of mayonnaise, the eggs are de-shelled, the yolk and albumen are separated. These separated constituents of whole real eggs are then re-combined with the following ingredients:

- Water
- Canola oil
- Maize (corn) starch
- Spirit vinegar
- Free range egg (2.5%)
- Modified maize starch
- Sugar, Salt
- Xanthan gum (stabiliser)
- Potassium sorbate (preservative)
- Natural mustard flavouring
- Concentrated lemon juice
- Calcium di-sodium [40] (EDTA) E 385 [41]
- Colour Paprika extract (E 160C [42])

This is the ingredient list for the *"light mayonnaise"* that we used to purchase from the local supermarket. Water is the main ingredient and the egg yolk itself comprises 2.5% of the total. So I wonder if the lemon juice is a concentrate or diluted form. Perhaps that is where some of the added water comes from? The other additives have been discussed elsewhere. For instance, xanthan gum, canola and corn starch in food processing is pretty much ubiquitous and is outlined in the *"Food Conspiracy"* book. Phrases including but not limited to "natural flavouring" [43] are designed to fool you. Chapter two outlines the practice of *"label washing"* and how it enables the industry to hide what it is doing to the food that most of us eat on a daily basis. As with the ice cream discussed in Chapter three, I fail to see how such a product can be referred to as mayonnaise. I know that mayonnaise is mainly a mixture of different oils and a few egg yolks, but 97.5% of the above mixture is not egg. Mayonnaise is never going to be a genuinely healthy option, all other factors considered; a classic mayonnaise is almost all oil. As a general rule of thumb, you use 2-3 eggs per 500ml of oil. The remainder is dashes of vinegar, salt, lemon juice, mustard and a clove or two of chopped garlic. Then the whole lot is mixed together as per the whisking instructions and there you have it. No water and none of the other additives. As for eggs themselves, the manufacturers can also choose from the array of egg mixes which are available for their perusal. If they don't fit specific requirements it is entirely possible for a new concoction to be developed. Such formulations are the mainstay of every ready-made quiche, sweet baked pastries, glazed pastry, meringue and sponge cake on the supermarket and convenience shop shelf. For really cheap processed foods eggs can be replaced wholesale. At the time of writing, the preferred egg substitutes are various types of whey proteins. They are derived from milk and aside from being cheaper than dried egg formulations, (the real reason for their use); whey proteins extend the life of a frozen food product by up to 18 months. Such realities make a *"best before date"* pretty much meaningless.

A natural flavouring may well have come from a plant, but it is certain to have been extracted with solvents and will not be limited to one flavour compound. If the label declares "natural mustard flavouring", "extract of XYZ", or "paprika extract" several chemicals are likely to fall under the heading. In general terms as long as the industry can say that the flavouring is not made in a laboratory and it is extracted from the plant, fruit or indeed animal in question, then it can be referred to as a *"natural flavouring"* (see chapter two). The probability that real paprika or mustard are present is going to be remote at best. The e numbers in the above list were put there by yours truly. I have only heard of potassium sorbate through my own winemaking. I only know what the initials EDTA mean because I have used it in the classroom and laboratory as a chemical indicator. Calcium di-sodium and other forms of EDTA are unlikely to have negative health impacts. The food industry uses this position to justify the presence of every single additive in the food it produces. Most additives are going to be safe for most people most of the time. The compounds calcium carbonate [44] (see chapter seven) and calcium sulphate (see chapter five) E 516 [45] have uses in food processing, over the counter medicines and as food supplements. Neither have any known toxic or negative health impacts. However, this is not the case with every substance we ingest. For instance, food dyes and colourants have been implicated in damage to human chromosomes and to the endocrine (hormone) transport system. These substances form one component of the label wash mentioned in chapter two. The food industry has learned its lessons from history (see chapter five) and no longer wilfully adds the more dangerous substances to the food we eat. However, it is not shy of cherry picking when it comes to public health. For instance, chapter five outlines how cured meats and similar foods are treated to prevent the growth of the microbe which causes the lethal syndrome we know as botulism. Sodium nitrite (E 250 [46]) and sodium nitrate work in an equivalent manner to the potassium salts mentioned in chapter five. They are highly effective in their stated preserving purpose, they are also used to add false colour to most processed and cured meats. Yet, both of these substances have been implicated in carcinogenesis (causing cancer). They are known to interact with stomach acids forming compounds called nitrosamines which are known carcinogens. A salt forms when non-metal atoms take the place of metal atoms in a given compound. The words sulphate, nitrate, carbonate or chloride

all denote compounds which are salts. The sodium salts do occur naturally in vegetables, but it is the synthetic forms that have been associated with pancreatic, colon and stomach cancers. These compounds are permitted for use in organic meats and the intensively produced variety. Both the organic [47] and non-organic sector agree that these compounds are safe. The organic sector will have strict limits on the amount of nitrate or nitrite that can be used. Whilst the intensive sector will operate under the banner of acceptable daily intake, this agency has a proven history of playing down the risk of food related disease, see chapter five. Both agencies have lobbied hard against banning the sodium salt compounds. Both agencies lobbied hard for the benefit of the producers. I use this example to demonstrate that not all is fluffy and benign in the land of organic food; it is a business just like any other. I also think this example underlines just how complex food issues truly are. However, Organic producers are generally not allowed to use synthetic forms of any substance. Plus, we ingest significantly more of the sodium compounds in their natural form in vegetables than we do the synthetic form in processed meats. The organic sector has openly admitted that natural forms of these compounds will make cured meats prohibitively expensive, hence an apparent approval for the synthetic form. The intensive sector will always opt for the cheaper synthetic and often oil based chemicals, whilst the organic sector generally does not. Organic or natural forms of the sodium compounds are derived from mineral or rock sources. It is also likely they can be derived from leafy green and other vegetables. Celery, for example, is a rich source of these sodium salts. However, as far as I can work out the UK organic sector is allowed to use synthetic forms of sodium nitrite and nitrate. Whether the synthetic forms are more dangerous than the natural form has yet to be established. If you are concerned on this matter, then the best course of action is going to be avoidance (see chapter three), because the compounds are not going anywhere and will be present in cured meats for the foreseeable future.

Depending on whose figures and exchange rate calculations you choose to believe, the food additives market is a huge global business with an annual turnover measured in hundreds of millions if not tens of billions of currency units. This also represents the foundation and crucial reality of the whole food additives business, it is absolutely first about profits and market share and absolutely last (if it is even mentioned) about health and nutrition. During the course of the research for this book and the Food Conspiracy volume, time and again the industry only talks about forecasts of growth and the particular additives and processing aids which are likely to drive it. The organic/permaculture sector uses entirely different language. And despite the sodium (and others not mentioned) contradiction mentioned above organisations who promote sustainable agriculture are the future, well, they better be, for all our sakes. Organisations have to make hard-nosed business decisions too. Perhaps if that sector had the financial support it so desperately needs (see chapter three) it would not need to make these decisions. The industry literature is brimming with predictions concerning percentage rates of growth in particular parts of the world and how foreign exchange rates may impact on that growth. Absolutely nothing is said about health, nutrition and the validity of the additive or production process in the first place. Now, you could be thinking, *"Ok, but it's a business, what do you expect?"* The answer has to be that this is an agency that exists to make a profit for itself and its shareholders and they will say and do anything in the achievement of that goal. The next chapter aims to demonstrate this point with reference to specific real world examples.

# Chapter Two: It's Not All About The Money Is It?

Until late 2013 I had no real understanding of how complex nutrition really is. If I'm honest whenever I heard the word I did have a tendency to roll my eyes and think of food fads, pretentious cooking and vacuous celebrity chefs. I am now absolutely disavowed of that position. The science of nutrition is just as complex, interesting and relevant to our survival and future as that of climate Earth and the other natural sciences. Since the mid-1990's I have vociferously campaigned against GMO's in agriculture and farming. I am aware of the political, social, environmental and economic aspects which thread through food and all other issues. Nevertheless, until a few years ago I had no real idea how the food manufacturers really operate. Intuitively and based on experience I knew it was not going to be a pretty sight. I was not surprised to learn how nefariously criminal the food processing industry is. The negative, system induced impact that our actions have, has a stratospherically high capacity to shock. The level of surprise is inversely related to the shock and this subject is no different. Yet, I had no knowledge of how interconnected food processing and big agriculture really is to other equally secretive transnational oligarchs. I had no real idea of how ugly and disgusting things are underneath the thin veneer of lies told by those who determine what is safe and good for us to eat. I was not looking, now I am. Speaking personally, I am bloody furious that I not only missed that particular boat but also that I didn't know the boat even existed. All of my writing on Vidda is a call for you to start looking too. You owe it to yourselves and you owe it to your children. I don't have children, but if I did, I would be even more upset and flat out furious about what has been done and continues to be done to our home than I already am. We live in a world that has been ravaged to the point of imminent collapse and one source of this ravishment is the perpetual global war we find ourselves in. I woke up to these realities in the late 1990's and it was the conflicts in Kosovo and Liberia that acted as catalysts. The debacles and destruction which went with Afghanistan, Chechnya and Iraq further showed the people who run our affairs for what they really are. We are ruled by a self-serving cabal of psychopaths who will sell the entire planet out to preserve their position. Unless we change the current self-destructive path, our current ridiculous position is the prologue for an impending conflagration which could well engulf us all in the very near future. Since the late 1990's I have believed that if our species and indeed life as we know it is to survive, three big and self-inflicted problems need to be resolved. And they need to be resolved yesterday. In no particular order these three global issues are:

- Nuclear power and nuclear weapons, i.e. nuclear issues.
- Climate change and all issues connected to it.
- The continuing and escalating global conflict we call World War Three and the depraved bonanza known as the armaments trade which is largely responsible for driving it.

In all three areas, I have seen absolutely nothing to compel a change of mind. On the contrary, my concerns and outright feelings of terror have intensified. In late 2013 I added food issues to this deceptively short list. The bottom line is that if we do not fix these issues we could well fall into a dark abyss of our own making. Given our all-encompassing and critically unstable global situation such a destination is ever more likely. Sadly, events since 2013 and in the run-up to autumn 2017 have dragged us all even further in the wrong direction. What is even worse is that so many people seem to be going along with it and/or somehow think we will be OK. At the very least we are destined for severe upheaval in the very near future that is if we do not change our ways pronto! As things stand our future is looking very bleak indeed. We are not on the cusp of some new golden age and the reader is well advised to get such nonsense out of their head right away. We are looking at total environmental, political, social and economic collapse. A worst-case scenario of **Permian Mass Extinction** [2] proportions truly is on the cards and we may not survive it. Too much is going wrong; too many **Rubicon's** [3] have been crossed and nothing like enough is being done to fix the catastrophe. In this arena *"something"* as they say *"is going to give"* and when it does...........what happens is anyone's guess. In our increasingly unstable, dictatorial and **anthroprocenic** [4] world, the chances are something or things will have already given, we just don't know it yet. This is not a message of doom and gloom; it is a frank and succinct appraisal of where we are right now in space and time. And when I last checked there is no planet B or worm hole through to the promised interstellar land. There are global, national and local solutions to these huge systemic global problems. What is missing is the political will and push from enough people in the western world (in particular) to make it happen. Having said all of that I am very pleased to write that in June 2017 enough people in the UK appear to have woken up to such realities. At the time of writing, I am optimistic that by the time you read this the current administration run by Theresa May and her new fundamentalist best friends will have been well and truly trounced. Assuming you have not made it already, you have a choice to make. As individuals and through established campaigning and/or political originations, we can start to repair the rot. We have every chance of not only surviving but creating a better world for all of us. After all, let us be honest, this one has cock-up and disaster written all over it, doesn't it? As an individual, one avenue toward creating a better future can be by starting to look at our food and what is being done to it. One essential step in that direction is to gain an appreciation of how the industry which makes most of our food really operates.

## Trade Shows and Business Deals

In 1986 an organisation called Food Ingredients Global (FIG) held its first trade show. FIG is but one of many industry trade fairs. The participants are looking for new ways to perfect existing food technology techniques and continually introduce new ones. The whole point is to improve and expand the utility of substances which already exist and introduce those which are just around the corner. FIG represents how intensive food production has been skewed from an agency that could easily produce healthy and affordable food for every person on the planet, into that which we see around us. FIG is but one representation of one of the biggest, darkest but cleverly hidden lies of the modern age. The lie being that food processing in its current form exists for the benefit of people, planet and community. FIG and their ilk perpetuate this particular lie. I'm not singling FIG out from equivalent organisations; they are all as contemptible as each other. Why the vitriol? Well, listen to the bilge that the links on the front page spew forth for a start. Listen and I mean really listen to how these people communicate, listen to the tone of the interviewers too. These people are not concerned with food in any meaningful sense; they are not concerned with food quality. They are business people and are only concerned with making as much money as possible. In this frame it does not matter how the money is made, but only that it is made. Have a quick look around the website and you will come across *"the complete package"* set of bullet points. I think it speaks for itself. There is no mention of *"health"* or *"nutrition"* but plenty is said about *"business solutions"* and *"specific markets"* along with *"the latest local and global innovations"*. The bi-yearly FIG event is a truly transnational undertaking. The last European exhibition took place in Paris over the first three days of December 2015. Each event attracts tens of thousands of delegates from the global food processing industry. The last FIG event took place in Frankfurt in November 2017. According to the FIG website, since 1986, over half a million people have come to view the latest offerings from the industry. Apparently, over 50 thousand delegates came to the last FIG meeting and it appears the November 2017 gathering attracted even more.

Billions of euros have been turned over since the first FIG trade fair and I wager none of it has been channelled into genuinely sustainable agriculture. If you take the time to peruse the FIG website another point soon becomes glaringly obvious. There is very little mention of food, or the food groups themselves. There is certainly no mention of vitamins, minerals, health or nutrition. Surely it would be reasonable, nay rational, even obvious, to expect such areas to be discussed. Yet, they seem only to be mentioned as a vehicle to carry out business. The obvious question is to ask why. Perhaps this statement from the FIG website will explain, *"it (FIG) brings together the world's leading food and beverage suppliers, research and development, production and marketing specialists and showcases the most diverse range of new and innovative ingredients and services".* To be absolutely crystal clear food, sustainability and agriculture are not the focus of these gatherings. From navigating the website, very little actual food appears to be on offer at the event. It is a three-day exhibition. The manufacturers are able to portfolio the totality of their latest additives, processing aids, preservatives and any other chemicals they choose, to the delegates who come to visit. From a skin deep perspective, this is not particularly problematic, after all, it is abundantly clear what the exhibition is all about. So, if you want to sample freshly prepared organic food (whatever that may mean) then perhaps you need to go to the nearest farmers market, instead of FIG. Sounds good to me, I know where I would rather be, clue, it's not at FIG. Unfortunately, it just isn't that simple. First, the exhibitions themselves are not open to the public. The organisers decide whether or not you can attend. Given that we are supposed to be the beneficiaries of the so called innovations on offer, I think this is more than a little contradictory. Secondly, to even be considered a delegate you must prove that you are employed in processed food and/or its manufacture. So, we have no real say in what goes on behind closed doors and you have to benefit from being at the gathering too. Behind the smiles and invitations to *"meet the team"* this is not a corporate jolly event. Here we are talking about hard-nosed business dealings and nothing else. This event and all the others like it are concerned with making as much profit as possible, period. Any prospective delegate will need to present a business case for being at the exhibition. Finally, before you even walk through the door you will have to book yourself a stand. Just don't be expecting to be talking about food when the sales rep contacts you.

We are all sold the lie of healthy food choices brought about by competition. Whether you believe the lie is down to you. As the industry views things, FIG and similar events are concerned with presenting the future of food technology. Innovation and technology as applied to food seem somewhat oxymoronic; I mean to say that I was not aware that food needs to be innovated or subject to the vagaries of profit driven technology. Food crops need to be grown sustainably and animals need to be reared responsibly. Clearly, in our world farmers, growers, gardeners and smallholders need a decent financial reward for their hard work. The soil has to be managed, maintained and respected, not treated like a bottomless resource. Beneficial traits in both food crops and livestock can be exploited and further developed but not at the expense of genetic diversity. In this circumstance innovation is a byword for profiteering. Based on what I have seen on the FIG website these and other related points are not even mentioned. FIG is a showcase for unnecessary food adulteration and not much else. At anytime, anywhere in the world, a FIG or equivalent event is happening or about to. Truly, these events have global implications for all of us. While they are allowed to happen there is no way that food production in its current form is going to stop. Intensive food processing and FIG events are part and parcel of the same coin. One cannot exist without the other. It is no coincidence that some of the core drivers and their subsidiaries behind GMO's are also present at FIG-esque events. The profits are too vast, the usual vested interests present and industrial cross-linkages are to be maintained as well as expanded. These events are not concerned with food per se. The overriding goal appears to revolve around extolling the virtues of a particular additive or production process. In about an hour of searching through the FIG website, I saw nothing about food, farming or agriculture. I don't think I even saw food as an essential part of our history, culture and evolution mentioned once. It is quite literally all about the *"additives"*, *"the processes"* and most important *"the money"*. Every other concern appears to be secondary in the minds of the organisers and by association those who attend. The combined buying power of the delegates and the organisations they represent is measured in billions of currency units. The exhibitors are going to want as much of that financial pie in their pockets as they can get. All the horse trading, sorry legitimate and professional business dealing happens outside of the public domain and so is free from any real scrutiny. Preceding the research for this book I didn't even know FIG existed. The secrecy draws me to one crystal clear conclusion. The industry would rather that you didn't know what it is up to and certainly does not want you asking questions about its activities. The industry will cite the all too common *"commercial confidentiality"* or *"restrictions under patent law"* for its stealth and secrecy. In reality, the stealth exists because the industry knows that people will be turned off by what it has to offer and how it operates. And that will translate into lost revenue and from their perspective that is intolerable. I have never attended such a gathering so I cannot say with absolute authority what they are like. However, whilst reading through the reports from those that have been in such places it becomes very clear as to whom I'm going to believe and trust. Clue, it's not the manufacturers or their motives! So the glaringly obvious question has to be *"what kind of innovations and processes are discussed at this and other similar gatherings?"* The examples outlined below will hopefully go some way to answering this question.

## Cheese, Glucono-Delta Lactone and Chymosin

Though my waistline would probably beg to differ I absolutely love feta cheese. Having lived in Southern Europe for several years I was able to try different types of fresh feta pretty much on tap. Now, that was a terrible job I can tell you, but hey ho! So, when I read of a cheese presented as *"feta with **glucono-delta lactone** [5] (GDL)",* I was automatically curious. GDL is a common food additive whose parent compound is a substance called **gluconic** [6] acid ($C_6H_{12}O_7$). It is an organic or carbon based acid and is found naturally in honey and fruits. It forms during ripening when glucose is oxidised, i.e. when glucose takes up oxygen atoms. As I write, the must which is fermenting into fruit wine is producing gluconic acid. The presence of this and other organic (carboxylic) acids will help the final wine take on a sharper, crisper taste. As a molecule and in alkaline conditions it is highly adept at hoovering up ions of calcium, copper, iron and aluminium. In food processing and manufacture this acid is designated as **E 574** [7] where it functions as a chelating (binding) agent and acidity regulator. Any substance which functions by keeping a food within narrow pH limits is defined as an acidity regulator. Acidity is measured by the pH scale. The scale runs from pH 1 which is most acidic to pH 14 which is most alkaline. The neutral point of the scale is pH 7, where pure water sits. The neutral point delimits the point between acidity and alkalinity. Gluconic acid is likely to have been produced *"by aerobic fermentation of a carbohydrate source",* almost certainly from genetically engineered corn. GDL production (**E 575** [8]) is likely to involve the use of genetically engineered microbes, which produce limitless quantities in bio-fermenters. In scientific language, GDL is an example of a cyclic ester of gluconic acid. It is produced by dehydrating gluconic acid. The dehydration leaves behind a white powdered crystalline solid. This method of production is being slowly superseded by methods which evaporate gluconic acid in a solution of dissolved glucose. As the *"Food Conspiracy book"* indicates glucose is increasingly being produced by means of genetically modified sugar cane and/or sugar beet. It is likely that the gluconic acid used to make GDL is likely to have come from genetically engineered **corn** [9] crops. Hence I can present another example of how biotechnology is becoming ever more entrenched into modern food manufacturing. Sadly, the number of individual examples is continually increasing and the entrenchment shows no sign of stopping.

Solid powdered GDL is highly soluble in water and when it dissolves the pH of the solution will decrease. For example, the acid inducing properties make it useful in maintaining the acidity of condiments and dressings. GDL works best when it is used in precise quantities and/or with other preservatives or antimicrobial agents. For instance, it works very well with sodium benzoate/**benzoic acid** [10] (E 210) (see chapter three) where the preserving properties of both molecules are enhanced. GDL is used in any circumstance where microbe growth at a lower pH is a possibility. Thus explaining why highly perishable foods are immersed in solutions of GDL and equivalent pH reducing substances. In traditional and organic circumstances feta cheese is preserved in a solution of brine or virgin olive oil. This is how the feta I am used to was available in southern Europe. All things being equal (which they are not due to price) I know which form I would prefer to eat, how about you, the reader? GDL functions by ensuring that potential microbes cannot turn a given food into a colony for themselves. Microbiology is the study of microbes. The discipline has established a direct relationship between water content and food spoilage. The more suitable moisture present, the more likely microbes are to set up shop and spoil food. The microbes care not one jot for the onset of spoilage, for them, it is party time. Acidity regulators help make it more difficult for microbes to spoil food. Feta is a highly perishable cheese and spoils within days even if it is wrapped and refrigerated. At this point, GDL and other acidity regulators come into proceedings. When added to any water based (aqueous) solution GDL will rapidly dissolve. As it dissolves it converts back into its gluconic acid precursor compound. The GDL/water solution begins to slowly increase in acidity, which in turn changes the taste of the cheese from sweet to acidic. The drop in pH also garners the preserving quantities mentioned above. According to the manufacturers, GDL produces a less acidic taste than citric and other acids. However, I would be willing to bet my last sheckles that citric acid is more expensive to produce than GDL. If a food preservation technique requires a slow decrease in pH the chances are that GDL has been employed. According to industry **sources,** [11] GDL can be injected straight into the cheese before final packaging. Then the cheese is stored in airtight containers. Before distribution and ultimate sale, the cheese is cut into bricks and then wrapped up in airtight plastic packets, with a little of the GDL solution to keep it preserved. GDL is a preservative added to processed feta cheese to extend its shelf and transportation life. Feta cheese is likely to have gone on a very long journey before it ends up in your fridge. The same will apply to pretty much any food that has been treated with preservatives. These substances are not added for our benefit. They are added to provide the illusion of freshness for as long as the producer can get away with under the law. Irrespective of the food in question, the primary reason for the preservation is to keep it as palatable as possible for as long as possible. The food is available for the longest possible time and that means increased profits throughout the entire resource and distribution chain. To the industry notions of food miles, health, nutrition and sustainability simply do not matter. Another source of profits is the multiple uses of the same substances in different industries. GDL is no exception. It is a hugely important molecule with various uses **outside** [12] of food processing. GDL is a Generally Regarded as Safe **(GRAS)** [13] (see chapter five) list substance. GDL is employed in skin treatment and **beauty** [14] products because it absorbs and retains water.

Chymosin is the workhorse enzyme for cheese manufacture. Up until the late 1980's, almost all rennet for cheese making was taken from the stomach lining of slaughtered calves. Until they are fully weaned milk is the principal food for calves. Cows are ruminant animals and if allowed to grow properly calves use rennet molecules to digest their mother's milk. Chymosin is the main molecule inside rennet which makes this digestion possible. It is an enzyme and it functions by catalysing the reactions which break down the proteins which make up the milk. Today, most chymosin is produced by the metabolism of genetically engineered microbes. Employing genetically engineered microbes which are stored in giant fermenters is **NOT** the same as developing a genetically engineered plant or animal. The essential difference between using a microbe to produce chymosin in cheese making or insulin in medicine and a GM crop or animal is very simple. Inserting the genetic material from the genes of the stomach lining of calves into a microbe so that it produces almost limitless quantities of chymosin represents a closed system. The microbe is stored in huge fermenters and the chymosin is syphoned off. There is no direct contact with the microbe and the outside world. A similar setup exists for insulin and dozens of if not hundreds of other beneficial biological molecules. With GM crops and animals there is direct interaction with the natural world. Expressing it alternatively, I have no problem with gene therapy (which is more regulated than GM crops and animals are), who in their right mind does? I also have no problem with the use of biotechnology to manufacture insulin or other hormones or the use of genetic engineering to produce useful enzymes. The pectolase I use to make wine has almost certainly come from a genetically engineered microbe. Discounting such arguments for now, (see chapter eight) the absolute and total reality of modern intensive hard cheese making is down to the action of enzymes, mainly chymosin. The gene technology was developed in the late

1980's. In 1990 the US FDA approved the use of genetically engineered organisms in hard cheese making. In the same year, the first cheese made with chymosin produced by means of genetic engineering began to sit on the supermarket shelf. In the 21st century, about 90% of all hard cheese is made in this way. Most of the cheese manufactured in the UK, EU and wider world has been made with chymosin from genetically engineered organisms. Clearly, unless you looked you wouldn't know it. I don't see *"made with GM chymosin/rennet"* on the label of the cheddar and parmesan which is in our fridge. I also cannot see in big block capitals the initials *"Preserved with GDL"* on packets of feta cheese. If you are not being told what is going into your food, or how it is made, the industry is willingly hiding something(s) from you. As a rational human being, it seems responsible to ask *"what else have they been doing behind closed doors?"* And it is from such questions that controversy and a lack of trust do germinate. Chymosin and other developments may not be problematic; for sure they may well produce benefits. However, I find it difficult with more than good reason to trust without question any activity carried out by the food processing and related industries. As chapter eight and the Introducing GMO's book imparts, genetically engineered crops and animals are a planet wide genetic disaster waiting to happen. I dread to think what the response from the food; biotech and chemical industries will be when things really start to go wrong with GM crops and animals, which they surely will.

Chymosin is the main coagulating enzyme found in rennet. It works by causing milk to aggregate or clump together into curds (the solids). The solid curds are separated from the liquid whey. The curds are used to make the final hard cheese. So far so good, after all, human beings have been making cheese for over 8000 [15] years. What is perhaps less well known is that food scientists can create the illusion of mature cheese in much the same way as they have been able to create the illusion of fresh bread by Chorleywood means (see the book "Food Conspiracy - What

48

Happened To Our Bread? - The Chorleywood Bread Process"). Depending on the type, traditionally matured hard cheeses stand for between 9 and 24 months. For even stronger cheese the time scale will be much longer, some cheeses are left for decades. This is not the case for the cheddar and parmesan in our fridge. I'm guessing it won't be for the equivalents in your fridge either. So what is the deal here? For these cheeses, various types of immature cheese are mixed together and then treated with lipase and protease enzymes. They catalyse the reactions which occur during natural maturation. The maturing time is cut to a few days. An equivalent *no time method* of producing mature cheeses as exists with Chorleywood bread making is occurring. This is not declared on the label. As far as this writing is concerned we have our first bona fide example of a food not being what it says it is on the label. Such cheeses really ought to be downgraded to something akin to a mature cheddar substitute or equivalent. Or it should clearly state matured with the use of XYZ enzymes. It really ought to be stated whether the cheese is a blend or not. Plenty of alcoholic drinks draw the distinction so why not with cheese and other foods too? The reader can be assured that hard cheese represents only the tip of a Larsen C sized iceberg. It is also one of the more relatively benign practices carried out during intensive food processing. Clearly making any cheese from offcuts or putting them to some other food related use is not the issue here. But offcuts which are stuck together and then matured by the action of enzymes is not to my mind a genuinely mature cheese. By all means use the offcuts in some capacity, perhaps by selling them as such. This is what happens with other foods, particularly cured meats, so why not with cheese? Palming off the excess blend and then processing them in the above manner should not be happening. Again the only reason such practices are carried out is for profit. If cheese making along with the entire food system were re-organised then genuine and affordable cheese would be the norm and not the exception. Once the required degree of artificial maturity has been achieved the cheese is gradually heated. The heating ceases the activity of the enzymes by causing them to denature.[16] The structure of the enzyme changes so that it can no longer carry out its aggregating function. As far as the industry is concerned, the enzymes are destroyed during the manufacture of a food which uses them. Enzymes are considered processing aids and **NOT** a designated ingredient. The manufacturer does not have to list **ANY** processing aids as ingredients, so they don't. The manufacturer does not have to declare:

- The enzymes used
- The quantity of enzymes used
- Why they are used
- How they convert an immature cheese into a mature form so quickly
- The type and source of the different blends of immature cheese which are converted

The use of enzymes in modern food production is not necessarily a problem, but these sorts of activities are designed to sell you a food which is not fit for purpose, whilst keeping the monetary cost to you as low as their bottom line will allow.

## Potato Protein Extracts (PPE's)

Here we are talking about a whole series of proteins which have been extracted from the **slurry** [17] produced by raw potato processing. Such activity is synonymous with the extrusion of cereal grains outlined in chapter one. This begs the glaringly obvious and recurring question, "*why is perfectly good fresh potato subjected to processing in the first place?*" Perhaps there are good solid reasons for converting fresh potatoes into a source of additives, but I have yet to come across one. The only reason these practices are allowed to happen is to make a profit. They serve no other purpose. By definition, there is no "*good solid reason*" for them to be happening. For such reasons and to absolve our household of some potato and corn related hypocrisy, our household intake of crisps, biscuits and tortilla chip has been curtailed to almost nothing. Not quite but nearly! On a related point, which crops up (pun intended) again in chapter three our household started making its own dips back in 2014! Anyway, back to PPE's, as with gluten proteins we are not discussing a single molecule. The PPE's represent another set of multi-use food additives, adulterants, preservatives and processing aids. We are discussing a whole family of proteins extracted from potato juice which fall under the heading **PPE**.[18] Various chemical processes take place to extract individual proteins and each can be isolated from its peers. Each individual protein is known as a Potato Protein Isolate (PPI). To my knowledge, the **production** [19] of PPI's began in Holland in 2007. Consequently, by **2008/9** [20] PPI's were part and parcel of sweet pastry making. PPI's are used to make sweetly baked confections including sponges, jellied fruit cakes and chocolate cakes. If a food is sweet and baked, it will likely contain PPI's. Alternatively, it is easier to say where PPI's do not exist as opposed to where they do. As a family of compounds, they have resided in the GRAS list (see chapters four and five) since March 2013. The PPI's do not appear to be particularly dangerous, but this is not the point. First, just because we have not come across any negative health impacts for any substance, does not mean we won't. Chapter four shows us that historically all sorts of substances that we now know are toxic have been used extensively to alter human food. The five year lag from PPI discovery to approval does not seem long enough to ascertain (or not) their toxicity. Having said that I don't think we will ever find that PPI's are toxic or dangerous. The same cannot be said for plenty of the other chemicals added to the food billions of human beings eat every day. And certainly not for the kind of substances mentioned in chapter five. Again, this is not the point. As shown in chapter one, notions of toxicity ignore or distract from the basic question as to why the extracts and isolates exist in the first place. It also ignores their potential for interaction with other substances. The PPI's were introduced by a Dutch company called Solanic Pharma-chem, itself a subsidiary of a larger concern called Avebe. Both company websites are listed at the end of this chapter. Avebe, the parent company produces specialist wheat, corn and tapioca starches for the following industries:

- **Processed food** [21]
- Textiles
- Paper
- Glue
- Animal Feed
- **Pet food** [22]

The processed food hyperlink takes you to an industry journal called *"Food Manufacture UK"*, whose website is also listed below. Although a cheerleader for the industry the site is a goldmine of information. I kid you not; you will never look at food in quite the same way again. I mention this in part because of the use of language employed by the website, which is identical to that presented on the FIG web site. In this particular example, the potato is *"humble"* and has had its *"potential unlocked"*. Well, I say there is nothing humble about a food which has been a staple food humanity for thousands of years. On that basis alone its potential has been well understood since the Neolithic Revolution. All the industry means by unlocking *"the potential"* of any food is separating out individual substances from a whole food and profiting from them. I say leave the PPI's where they are (inside the potato) and make sure everyone eats the glorious and amazing spud, pomme de terre, y patatas, as it should be eaten. As Sam in the *"two towers"* states with great animation, you can mash them, boil them, chip them, and you can roast them too. Well, he says something like that and the point I think has been made, so it's close enough! Potatoes do not need to be turned into an off white coloured slurry with a slightly blue tinge and be reduced to a collection of individual molecules. Potatoes are meant to be eaten whole as they have been for thousands of years. The very same isolates which are likely to be present in sweet baked foods are also likely to be present in the products of the above-mentioned industries. The use of PPI's is not limited to sweet bakes so it seems sensible to ask *"where"* and *"why"* PPI's are present in the food we eat. The *"where"* part is listed below:

- In **gluten** [23] free sweet and savoury bakes.
- As a substitute for animal proteins, any *"ready meal"* which is vegan or vegetarian is likely to contain PPI's.
- In alcoholic and non-alcoholic drinks.
- In **sports** [24] and energy drinks.
- In foods and supplements presented as a method to improve **cardiovascular** [25] health. The industry holds that the amino acid count is higher in PPI's than other protein sources. So they are touted as being beneficial for people embarking on a health and fitness programme.
- In substitutes for dairy products, particularly milk, cheese, butter and cream.

According to the industry, there is very little to distinguish a cake baked with the *"traditional"* ingredients and an equivalent baked with PPI's. By a stunning coincidence, the potato substitute just happens to be cheaper than the ingredients that have been used in the past, which explains the *"why"* of PPI's. The FIG website absolutely demonstrates that developments like PPI's are not unique or special case examples. They are part and parcel of how modern intensive food production is organised. The entire industry is built around making a profit from food manufacturing and processing thereof. These gatherings exist to celebrate how the profit objective is achieved. The industry believes, or states, it is beneficial to remove as much milk protein as it can from the entirety of production of all baked foods. The manufacturers want to increase the portion of protein used in *"aerated cakes"* (sponge cakes to you and I) and replace it with

PPI's. It would appear that they have been successful in this particular endeavour. Before 2007 between 2 and 4.5 percent of all the proteins found in sweet bakes came from milk protein. In late 2017 the figure is less than 1 percent with the difference being taken up by PPI's. According to the industry, there has been no discernible loss in quality, taste or functionality (whatever that means) as a result of the swap. This may well be the case, but writing personally I don't care. The fundamental point in all of this has been ignored and circumvented. Modern sweet bakes are light years away from those that my grandmother used to make. The ingredients used to make them would have been given short shrift by my grandparents as well. None of this is supposed to matter to us and from the industrial perspective, the PPI's also have another clear cut benefit. I wager the following sentence is the real reason for their continued existence.

They are known to intensify the flavour of other ingredients. This means food scientists are able to tweak a given food so that an individual PPI can be matched to a particular flavour, allegedly improving the taste of the food in question. Well, you call me Mr Picky if you will, but I prefer my food to be as fresh and unprocessed as possible. So, how about this radical idea, how about growing and distributing the food we eat properly? Then perhaps it would not need improving. Under the banner of "label washing" (see below) and under certain circumstances, with PPI's less artificial flavourings are necessary. This does not mean the food is going to be any fresher, healthier or nutritious. It does not mean that fewer preservatives, processing aids or indeed artificial flavours themselves will be used. It means that different amounts of different additives will be used in conjunction with a given set of, or with individual PPI's. The total quantities of additives do not change, merely their combinations. The PPI's represent another facet of the label washing mentioned below. In specific processes, the PPI's also act as excellent **emulsifiers.** [26] This hyperlink takes you to a website called food navigator, another industry mouth piece which is also a treasure chest of information. The website is also listed below. In this PPI example, all that has happened is a substitution of additives already present for another set of chemicals extracted from a nominally unprocessed food source, i.e. the potato tuber itself. To my mind, neither should be in the food in the first place. On top that any reduction in the use of artificial flavourings as a result of using PPI's will only increase profits for the manufacturers. You will not see a reduction in the costs of your food shopping. In a post-EU membership Britain the opposite is likely to occur. We can all expect the manufacturers to use the divorce from the EU as an excuse to increase their already bloated profits. In addition to any food price increases, we can also expect a further watering down of current food regulation if the current Brexit direction continues. I am no fan of the EU, but Brexit is a huge mistake that one way or the other is going to cost those who voted for it and the equivalent millions who didn't dear. Even a cursory look at the political situation in the UK as of late 2017 should make that point beyond obvious.

**Butter Buds**

Whilst researching the above section I came across a granulated, cholesterol free butter substitute called **butter buds**.[27] The butter buds website is also listed below. It is filled with phrases which impart that their product *"provides functional concentrated dairy flavours to global food manufacturers"*. And they use *"proprietary enzyme technology"* (PET) to provide the necessary flavours. PET means that a company *"owns"* the enzyme and any applications which use it. Butter buds are produced by the action of enzymes which release the strong flavour chemicals found in the fats of dairy products. The *"butter buds"* process and enzymes themselves are still patented and so *"owned or appropriated"* by a US concern called the Cumberland Packing Corporation (CPC), whose website is also listed below. It should not surprise the reader to find that the CPC also own the butter buds corporation. The reader should be assured that the technology will be in use elsewhere, and will be providing CPC with additional revenue. However, there is zero obligation on the CPC to declare this interest. According to the butter buds website:

- Butter buds dairy concentrates create better tasting and healthier foods, whilst reducing costs. They do not say what they mean by costs (I assume cash), neither do they say who benefits from the reductions (I assume them, not us).
- Butter buds provide the natural attributes of cream and cheese.
- Butter buds are heart healthy ingredients adding negligible fat and cholesterol to the diet. The implication from this is that somehow processed butter substitute is better for you than real unaltered butter.

According to the manufacturers, butter buds are *"an enzyme-modified encapsulated butter flavour that has as much as 400 times the flavour intensity of butter"*, at a fraction of the cost of the real thing. I wonder with reference to the chapters on aspartame (six) and artificial sweeteners (seven) if the reader has heard this kind of drivel before? Personally, I'd rather have **un-altered** [28] churned cream or whole milk on my toast! That is milk which has come from cows which are outside, fed on grasses and has not been filled with antibiotics and where the animal is not suffering from mastitis. Butter Buds also contains maltodextrin produced from corn oil, they are almost certainly going to contain **derivatives [29] from genetically modified corn**. The corn itself would have been grown in a field which is part of the environment around us and is, therefore, interacting with the biggest open system known to us, the planet itself. The notion that ordinary butter, from grass fed cows, is better for you, as part of your healthy well balanced diet, is completely absent from the website. The CPC manufacture a range of artificial sweeteners and salt substitutes which contain no sodium. The business **relationship** [30] between the CPC and butter buds appears to be very cosy indeed and will be in place for several decades to come. For reasons of *"commercial confidentiality"* the processes and substances which make the butter buds process possible will not be in the public domain until the patents run out. Likely, the same technology will be used by CPC and the organisations which fall under its umbrella. Butter buds were developed in 1979. In the US they have become pretty much ubiquitous in dairy food processing. The CPC has links to over 500 food processing firms and this number will only continue to increase. At the time of writing, the corporation is trying to aggressively move into the processed cheese market. Consequently, with such operators making further inroads into cheese making we can expect even more of the practices outlined above.

## Tomatoes, Starches and Modifications

The "Introducing GMO's book" gave an overview of the total fiasco represented by the genetically modified *"flavr-savr tomato"*. Once that particular section has been read and assimilated it is clear that even on its own terms, this early foray into GM foods was a total fiasco. On its own terms does not mean those standards that a rational construct would seek to attain, namely sustainability and productivity. On its own terms means that the flavr-savr tomato did not deliver the financial goods and that genetically engineered tomato itself failed to live up to anything like expectations. I am not surprised to read of new tomato enhancing substances being developed and of new varieties of genetically engineered tomato. [31] Once again we are supposed to believe that such developments are occurring for our collective benefit. Not as people or human beings you understand, but as *"consumers"*. We are also supposed to believe that the lessons from past mistakes have been learned. Except they are not mistakes, the consequences are the result of deliberate policy. We are also supposed to believe that plants engineered to produce extra nutrients or even medicines are going to improve our health. They won't, quite the opposite. There are much simpler and less expensive ways to improve the health of all the peoples of planet Earth. One sweepingly obvious idea might be to provide and fund healthcare, free for every single person alive on the Earth at the point of need. A second idea could be to grow and provide healthy, home grown organic/permaculture food and organise its distribution. A good start to achieving such lofty objectives would be to stop processing food solely to make a profit. GMO's represent the status quo with highly likely and dangerous and irreversible genetic consequences to boot. A global *"dig for victory"* programme (for want of a better expression) would seem to be a better idea than what we have right now. Right back to the subject in hand! In a FIG context, the industry sponsored developments are supposedly going to improve the thickness and appearance of different tomato pastes and sauces. If you need to thicken a tomato sauce so that it doesn't leak out of its container. Or, if you wish the sauce to appear glossy for longer even after it has been opened, then two possible solutions present themselves:

- Microlys [32]: A speciality potato based starch which thickens liquids and garners a smooth shiny surface. It is a stabilising compound. Coincidentally, microlys is cheaper than other forms of starch.
- Pulpiz [33]: A pulp extender manufactured by Tate and Lyle which gives the appearance of ordinary tomato sauce.

Both products are based on a collection of molecules known as modified starch [34] and they are covered by the numbers E 1400 to E 1450 inclusive [35]. Starch is a natural polymer molecule composed of individual glucose molecules. As with the cellulose outlined in chapter one, each glucose molecule is bonded to its neighbour by a structure called a glycosidic bond. Starch molecules are insoluble in water and are a source of chemical energy for plants. Through another chemical sleight of hand, the food industry is able to present *"modified starches"* as natural starches. As far as the industry is concerned there is no chemical difference between *"natural"* starch and *"modified"* starch. In this frame, *"modified"* has nothing to do with genetic engineering or GM crops, unless the starch itself is derived from a GMO! Here, a starch has been modified if the chemical structure, bonding and/or orientation of the atoms which compose the molecule itself are changed. The modification techniques employed by the food manufacturers are designed to change the physical properties and chemical structure of the starch to garner some beneficial outcome for the industry. For instance, the water solubility can be enhanced such that the gelling or thickening properties of a base solution can be improved. For example, acetylated di-starch adipate (E 1422 [36]) has been chemically reacted with acetic and then adipic acid [37] (E 355 [38]) to improve its capacity to retain water. Adipic acid is necessary for the manufacture of nylon and is relatively rare in nature. For food manufacturing, the main source is from sugar cane or sugar beet. So, the adipic acid is likely to be derived from GM crops. Processes which require the retention of water are likely to employ chemically altered forms of starch. Plus, it is often necessary to ensure that the starch can withstand reductions in pH, i.e. increases in acidity. The point on GMO's is clear and present. It is entirely possible that acetylated di-starch adipate is derived from GM corn. The same is likely to be true for other modified starches. The now defunct, but formerly EU funded GMO compass website clearly state that the GM status of di-starch adipate *"may change in the near future"*; just don't expect the biotechnology industry to tell you about it. However, the food industry does seem to be sticking with non-GM [39] starches. How long for, is an open question!

You will see modified starch listed as an ingredient in foods ranging from gravy granules and cake mixes to salad dressings and fillings for pies and pastries. Collectively, the cellulose molecules mentioned in chapter one are all modified forms of starch. The modifications are also important for holding the starch polymers together. The molecules are subject to physical stresses, meaning heat and pressure changes as well as chemical stresses as they travel through a given production process. Starch grains can be altered by chemical and physical means. In the future, I will likely be able to add by *"genetic means"* and make a complete negative troika. Currently, the label only has to impart that the starch has been modified, which produces the meaningless phrase *"modified starch"*. The industry is under no obligation to declare what has happened, why it has happened, how it happens or the chemicals or process involved in the modification itself. So, you are unlikely to see pre-gelatinised or physically modified starch on the ingredient label. Needless to say, there is no associated obligation on the manufacturer to declare whether the starch itself is from a genetically modified source. Having said that, some manufacturers are promoting the starches they make as being from non-GMO [40] sources. Before we start congratulating such organisations we have to understand that their understanding of GM free is not the same as mine or anyone else who thinks that GM fee means exactly that. It is perfectly legal for any company to say its product contains no GMO's when the food in question can contain them. For instance, in the EU a food can be labelled as being GM free as long as it contains less than 0.9% GMO. [41] In the future I expect the modified starches to include those which have been made through genetic engineering. The modified starches are employed so that the minimum possible quantity of other ingredients can be employed in the pursuit of making the food itself. Many of the *"modified starches"* are also employed by the chemical and pharmaceutical industries. A further example is a class of compounds known as *"co-texturisers"*, and pulping [42] agents which are broadly similar to the modified starches outlined above. However, these starches are classified as *"functional native starches"* but are often labelled as starch. 43 Some of these starches are certified for organic processed organic foods provided they are not derived from GM sources.

## Sealing, Citric Acid, Labels and Extracts

Previous to our ancestral discovery of fire, our predecessors learned how to organise themselves. One devastating consequence of this organisation was the extinction levels of hunting of various species of mega fauna 44 which used to abound the surface and seas of the Earth. With the harnessing of fire came the final extinction of many of these great animals. The reasons for their demise are myriad and complex. Hunting by hominid animals is only part of the story, but rapid environmental changes also contribute to the loss of the big animals. Human beings have been preserving and storing foods since the Neolithic revolution. For instance, we are all familiar with the use of salt and smoke to respectively preserve food and enhance its flavour. Indeed, the wine I enjoy making uses Campden tablets as a source of sulphur dioxide ($SO_2$) to increase the acidity of the must, thus making it uninhabitable for microbes. The modern food industry has taken these and other necessary steps to an entirely different and in many respects undesirable level. FIG promotes the use of a solution called *"Nature Seal"* (website listed below). Nature seal will be one of many preserving solutions available at the next FIG event. It contains citric acid and other substances which add weeks to the shelf and transportation life of fruits and vegetables. Citric acid is doing its job in our latest batch of wine; it is stopping the peeled, chopped and pulped apples from turning black. The citric acid is preventing the fruit from oxidising. The acid itself came from a couple of squeezed lemons and half a lime. However, this kind of natural preservation is not what nature seal and equivalent solutions are concerned with. Once treated with nature seal solutions fruits and vegetables do not display the tell-tale signs of ageing and oxidation. Potatoes do not turn black, apples and pears do not turn brown, bananas do not become blotchy, citrus fruits do not collapse, and melons don't begin to leak. All of this is designed to give the appearance of freshness; the key word here is *"appearance"*. According to the nature seal web site, we as *"consumers"* (when last I checked I was a person) are supposed to be excited about the prospect of *"products"* which *"maintain their fresh qualities"*. Well, I'm not; I feel somewhat repulsed. For more information feel free to *"click on the consumer link on the left for more information"*. So if you love the idea of eating foods which have been treated so that *"they look good and taste fresh for up to two weeks"*, you know where to go. As with the enzymes used in the Chorleywood Bread Process (CBP), the substances which provide the illusion of freshness are termed processing aids. We already know that means the manufacturer does not have to declare the preserving agents have been used. It also means that there is no compulsion to inform that the food itself could be up to a month old. This is not fresh food, it has been preserved and the two positions are not identical, or (as the industry prefers to phrase it) substantially equivalent. We are told by those who profit from such developments that they are beneficial to us. They give us more choice and keep the food we eat affordable. For instance, nature seal preservation is touted as a mechanism to help curtail the appalling waste of food which occurs both domestically and in the catering/hospitality industry. The logic presumably being, that if food is preserved for longer, less of it will be bought. I would argue that a better strategy is to roll out *"Food for Life Partnerships"* (website listed below) and their equivalents on a national scale and have equivalent initiatives occurring globally.

Amongst its many activities the food industry has embarked on a strategy it calls *"Operation Clean Label"* (website listed below). This is nothing more than an additive wash campaign. It is directly comparable to the *"green washing"* conducted by businesses wishing to demonstrate their non-existent environmental credentials. The global clean label campaign is designed to remove the more obviously concerning additives and substitute for others which sound much less dangerous or can be framed as beneficial. The names have been changed [45] to protect the guilty, so no change there then! Or alternatively, it's about cleaning the *"label"* and not cleaning *"the food"*. Some additives and improvers have been replaced for the *"right"* reasons, that is, because they are known to do harm to the body and/or the environment. However, one can be assured that the food industry fights tooth and nail against such developments, especially if they affect their profit margin. We are concerned with an industry which qualifies its standards in terms of "limits of acceptability".[46] A limit is set based on what the industry has determined to be a safe level for a given substance. Two points present themselves. The manufacturers determine what goes into the food and how it is labelled (if at all). Second the manufacturers through the science they fund determine how much of a given substance is permitted in a given food stuff. The industry demonstrates stratospherically high levels of inertia when it comes to making meaningful change to how it operates, especially if the change impacts on its bottom line. The pursuit of profit supersedes all other concerns. If the manufacturer does not feel that it can pass on the cost of a change to the retailer, so that it is paid by us the public, then they will resist that change for as long as possible. At every possible opportunity, they resist paying for it out of their own bank balance. In such a situation the only recourse is to opt for cheaper additives and/or change the names of the substances in question. The idea is to wash away the perception and understanding that some of the many thousands of different additives may be dangerous to human health and/or the wider environment. How else do we explain the following example points:

- Why are the names of e numbers substituted for the name of the substance the number denotes? Because carmoisine [47] sounds much better than E 122.[48]
- Why do the food labels proudly declare virtually fat-free or

99 percent pure? Because you are not supposed to think about what is really in your food. We should be asking what is meant by pure and what is in the 99 percent portion. The same goes for statements which declare fat, sugar, gluten or lactose free.

- Identical points can be levied concerning *"no artificial colours"* and *"no artificial flavours"*. The reason for these phrases and what they really mean is discussed below.
- Why are chemical sounding names and any term that might shout *"artificial"* substituted for more benign sounding names? Because cellulose gum is more attractive than *carboxy-methylcellulose.* (See chapter one)
- Carmine, pink colour, cochineal or a number, for instance, E 120 [49] are used to cover up the real source of the substance in question. For instance, carmine is a pigment extracted from an insect species called Dactylopius coccus.[50] It takes about 100,000 insects to produce about a kilo of carmine.

The manufacturers know that if they were clear about such realities, that the *"yuck"* factor (see below) would likely provoke a negative reaction. I would bet now that if the reader were to check their diet and it had E 120 in it, you would be a little upset, especially if you have opted for a vegan or vegetarian diet. On the other side of the coin, we must realise that if we want to eat more *"natural"* ingredients then these sorts of pigments are going to present in the diet. We would then have to look at the ethics and reasons for using such substances in human food. At points such as this, the arguments for adopting a vegan, vegetarian or plant based diet come to the fore. If using such ingredients has adverse impacts on the natural world than I argue their use ought to be banned outright.

In the same vein, if you saw "rosemary extract" [51] as a listed ingredient you would naturally assume that the extract came from the rosemary herb. I know I did! Alas, you would through no fault of your own be wrong, like I was. As I made clear in the introduction I am no expert on any of this and I really am following my nose as I put all of this together. So, what is the story with the extracts? Well, rosemary extract is an anti-oxidant [52] which contains combinations of carnosic acid [53] (also found in other herbs) and dozens of other anti-oxidant [54] chemicals. In food processing, anti-oxidants slow down the rate at which foods spoil. They are a tried and tested method to extend the shelf and transportation life of a given food. For human and animal metabolism the benefits [55] of ingesting such compounds in their natural form are clear and present. For instance, alpha-pinene is one active ingredient of the rosemary herb and is a known anti-inflammatory. Extract of rosemary is denoted by the number E 392 and it is used in many processed foods including [56] spreads and butter. As with equivalent synthetic compounds (E300 to E321) [57] extract of rosemary prevents food from spoiling by preventing reactions with oxygen in the air we breathe. The anti-oxidant property is made possible by carnosic acid and rosemarinic acid. In this form, the acids will not add or enhance the flavour of any food they are added to. The acids have been extracted by use of chemical solvents or they may be synthetic copies of the natural form. The anti-oxidant compounds have unfamiliar chemical names, for instance, butyl-hydroxy-anisole [58](BHA/E 320) and butyl-hydroxy-toluene [59] (BHT/E 321). Many compounds which are *"good"* for us have such names. The naming of such compounds may appear confusing, but they exist so that chemists can precisely organise, name and classify the hundreds of millions of different compounds around us. In themselves, chemical names and the compounds are nothing to worry about. Some compounds with long names are beneficial, but BHA has been noted as *"reasonably anticipated to be a human carcinogen"* if the dose is high enough and regular enough. BHA may or may not be a carcinogen, but it is certainly one of those substances (along with BHT) which are regularly assessed. The 2011 EFSA acceptable limit for BHA is 1.0mg/kg of body weight per day. BHA is used extensively by the food processing industry because it can withstand heat and physical stress much more readily than other anti-oxidants [60]. BHT has no known potential carcinogenicity, but aside from that, it has equivalent utility to BHA. Both compounds are found in dozens of foods. They appear to complement each other in their anti-oxidant activity. They are also used extensively as solvents, in petro-chemicals and paints, the wider chemical industry, rubber manufacture, beauty products and in pharmaceuticals. Little wonder, that substances labelled as rosemary or other extract, appear more attractive than synthetic and possibly carcinogenic compounds. It would also explain why some manufacturers under specific circumstances are removing BHT and BHA from their manufacturing processes. For instance, The General Mills Company has removed [61] BHT from its US cereal manufacturing wing of operations. The replacement anti-oxidant molecules are the extracts of rosemary and other herbs mentioned in this section. The two basic questions which run throughout this book, once again present themselves. First, *"why is the substance necessary at all"*? And second *"why is the process itself occurring"*?

The number E 392 refers to any extract of rosemary which is then used as a food additive. Any substance which can be extracted from the rosemary herb can be referred to as E 392. This begs the obvious question, *"how can the industry label a group of additives as extracts of anything and then indicate them as one substance?"* In one word the answer is chemistry. Once it is known which chemicals in a given plant garner a particular property that substance can either be extracted directly or a synthetic form is manufactured. In manufacturing, we are talking about generic copies of *"natural chemicals"* which are produced by the *"food wing"* of a given chemical company. With extraction, the desired ingredient is taken by chemical means from the plant itself. Normally, the plant is pulped and then solvents are used to dissolve the target molecules. Then the solvent is evaporated off, leaving solid crystals which are then purified further. Plus, only the active compound and none of the flavour, texture, smell or taste of the plant is used. Next, the extract is converted to a convenient form for transport, normally a crystalline powder. Such processing converts rosemary or other whole foods into a solid concentrate of a specific substance. I have just read this section out to a few friends and the response, *"Mmmmmm yum yum"* was dripping in its sarcasm. Then the extract is sold on to the manufacturers who use it as they see fit. If you see *"extract of......."* on the label, the connection of the extracted substance to the plant it came from is as strong as humanities connection to life on Mars. Such that it doesn't exist!

## Cysteine

The food industry is well aware that perception is everything. It will say and do anything to minimise the "yuck factor" [62]. Otherwise known as the *"wisdom of repugnance"* or the *"evolved disgust response"*, the yuck factor elicits an emotional response to abnormal, new, strange, unfamiliar and potentially dangerous situations. The yuck [63] factor exists for a reason; it enables us to act in our own best interest and make the best judgement in a given situation. It is also related to that other evolved self-preservation mechanism known as *"the fight or flight response"*. We ignore, deny and suppress such emotional responses at our peril. Human beings have different responses to a given situation. So, the response, or not, is very much in the emotional make-up of the beholder. These and other emotional responses thread into your own individual barometer of acceptance. My barometer is somewhere just above the surface of the Marianas Trench, the deepest point in the crust of the Earth. My barometer is approximately eleven kilometres beneath the surface of the Pacific Ocean. At the other end of the scale, other people have a barometer which activates near the outer reaches of the Martian atmosphere. The Yuck response, like the fight or flight response, or that surge of *"uh oh this is not right"* has evolved to keep you safe. It should always elicit a common sense response, especially when we consider our food choices. For example:

- Food A is grown *"organically"* distributed with the minimum of packaging and additives and a fair share of your hard earned goes to the cooperative farm the food came from.
- Food B is grown on an intensive farm and sprayed liberally with pesticides, has enough food miles to get you to the moon and back and is packaged excessively. The price paid to the grower is set by the supermarket.
- Food C is grown as food B but has also been genetically engineered with a gene from a species of frog to make it resistant to infection.[64]

To put it bluntly and all things being equal, the yuck factor and basic common sense should compel you to choose option A. However, in the real world things are anything but equal and the obvious becomes impossible for most of us. You don't need a degree in economics to realise that if food A is the most expensive by default you will opt for one of the others. If you have ever tried to balance the books as an impoverished student or had to choose between baked beans or bread because you can't afford both, the notion of buying organic food is laughable. So assuming that cash is no object, the simple question to ask is *"which would you buy?"* the answer has to be food A. Both the industry and the powers that be know this reality to be self-evident to the point of fact. Both agencies know that given a straight and fair choice we (the public) will always opt for the healthy [65] and additive free alternative [66] every time. Or in more familiar terms, which would you prefer *"a hearty meal cooked to perfection with locally sourced ingredients?"* or *"a ready meal for one, from the freezer section in a budget supermarket?"* Yes, the answer is indeed obvious. The food industry employs every strategy it can to project perceptions of quality, health, nutrition, wholesomeness and even love as attributes it wants you to associate with its products and the additives which lace them. All of it at a price you can afford and all of the adulterations [67] carried out for your benefit. The industry does not want you to pay too much attention to how you may feel about what you are eating. This is one reason for their focus on price and shouts of choice from its advertising. The industry wants you to be assured that all is well; perhaps the next example may give another reason for their position.

The number E 920 is discussed in some detail in *"the Food Conspiracy book"*. The number identifies a substance called l-cysteine, [68] which breaks down into a non-essential amino acid called cysteine. A non-essential amino acid is one which human beings and other animals can manufacture themselves, normally in the liver. In our context cysteine functions by removing oxygen from the food in question, it is also an anti-oxidant. In human metabolism, cysteine is necessary for the manufacture of a substance called glutathione. This molecule is particularly effective in repairing free radical damage to cells. L-cysteine also partially composes the chemical make-up of L-cysteine hydrochloride (E 920) and [69] L-cysteine hydrochloride monohydrate (E 921). In mammals, cysteine is a key component of a structural protein called keratin, which is found in the hair and nails. Similarly, in birds, it composes up to 12% of the feathers and egg shell. Throughout the biosphere, l-cysteine is a hugely important structural molecule. Up until very recently the main source of cysteine was the hair and feathers of slaughtered animals. In the modern world, cysteine is produced by chemical means by, amongst others, a company called Ajinomoto. [70] They are based in China; where about 80 percent of all synthetic cysteine is manufactured. Where the l-cysteine comes from [71] is a question whose answer is wide open to debate. In the past, The Ajinomoto Company has claimed [72] that Cysteine from human and animal origin has found its way into the human food chain. I am no cheerleader for Ajinomoto; apart from any other points until putting this book together, I had never heard of them. That should again indicate something about the secrecy around sourcing additives and how the whole industry operates. Well, it did to me! Perhaps it's a demonstration of my total cynicism and complete lack of belief concerning how *"the world is run"* but I would not put it past the food industry to use cysteine from human and/or animal sources. After all, even a cursory glance at the foods scandals in just the UK show that the industry will cut corners and keep its operations under a veil of secrecy. The industry will absolutely keep this secrecy maintained for as long as possible, especially if it results in increased profits. The 2014 horsemeat furore is but one demonstration of how the industry keeps its operations well and truly hidden from the public domain. [73] Human hair is 20 percent cysteine, which makes us one of the most concentrated sources of cysteine in the animal kingdom. In our world, all that you see around you, including you is a commodity to be exploited. It is not far-fetched [74] to suggest that cysteine from human beings would be a convenient and cheap raw material. That being said, even by the benthic (bottom dwelling) standards of today's maladjusted world, using cysteine of human origin is still going to be illegal. Leaving sourcing questions aside for a moment, the industry maintains that L-cysteine hydrochloride is destroyed by heat. So, it joins the hundreds of other substances which sit under the heading processing aid. Again, the manufacturers can avoid declaring the existence, source or production of any l-cysteine hydrochloride and its derivatives. Equally, it would be wilfully duplicitous to suggest that Ajinomoto were making the above claims for the *"right"* reasons. More likely such claims are made for *"commercial"* reasons. This also means that such claims may be unfounded, but on the other hand, they may not, the point is we cannot check. Such realities ought to make us wonder about the entirety of additives and their derivatives which are in the food we eat. To this writer, it all seems very grubby, somewhat vulgar and very yucky indeed.

The industry driven clean labelling initiative is not about providing fresh unprocessed and natural ingredients for human beings. Clean labelling is another strategy the industry employs to further shield its activities and pretty much develop and/or exploit any substance it chooses. There is no statute compelling the industry to inform the population (i.e. us) about such developments. Under current EU labelling law, we are supposed to trust the entirety of ingredients as being safe both for ourselves and the environment around us. I wonder in a post-Brexit Britain how much further this trust will be undermined in the pursuit of profits? The reader should be assured that the industry will present scientific data explaining that the level of a given substance or family of chemicals is well below that which is toxic. In many cases, this is undoubtedly true but equally, there are dozens if not hundreds of examples where the opposite is the case. The phrase *"acceptable limit"* [75] is just one example of how the industry assesses the suitability of a given substance. The US food industry uses GRAS and for GMO's you will see my personal favourite *"substantial equivalence"* [76]. The last phrase represents a position held by the food industry and the industries it is connected to. Namely, they will impart that no difference exists between *"synthetic"* and *"natural"* compounds. It will say that the additive concerned operates in isolation from others which may be present. Clearly, we do not eat any additives in isolation from the others. You don't need a degree in science to appreciate that, all you need to do is take a look at the ingredients listed on the foods in your kitchen. The potential for a very real additive "cocktail effect" [77] is not an issue that the industry is willing to discuss, let alone thoroughly research. When we consider that many of the additives found in the food we eat are found in plenty of non-food products, I think this is a grotesquely irresponsible and downright criminal position to take. For instance, research abounds which indicates that different combinations of different additives can and do have adverse effects [78] on the metabolism of human beings. On an individual and acceptable limit basis, it may well be true that limit X of substance Y is safe. By the same token if the research does not qualify itself by imparting that substance X is not ingested in isolation from other substances, then assertions of safety cannot remain unchallenged.

**Food Ingredients Global is part of Big Agriculture**

Intensive scale food processing is an integral part of a global construct known as *"big agriculture"*. FIG is merely one component of a very large machine. FIG and equivalent events are not accessible for most of us so we have no real say in what is discussed, what is decided or what business decisions are taken. Most of us have no choice but to visit the friendly face of this nefarious oligarchy, AKA the local supermarket. This friendly face is the front end of a resource chain that often extends to locations thousands of miles away. Where else do those pretty little packets of vegetables come from? Where else do the substances so many of our *"sophisticated and precision made modern"* food choices contain come from? The entire *"big agriculture"* construct exists to make money, wherever and however it can. Greed is absolutely hardwired into its operations, from supermarket shelves all the way through the resource chain. Despite what the advertising and PR tells you, absolutely nothing is allowed to get in the way of generating cash.

We now have a ridiculous (and criminal) situation whereby the food manufacturers can combine hundreds if not thousands of ingredients which are simply not found in nature. A dearth of effective legislation, let alone a desire to enforce it means there is practically no regulatory framework as to how the combinations are employed. It is these combinations and their applications which are discussed at FIG. The standard response to these concerns runs along the lines of *"additives pose no risk to human health"* when they *"are ingested in normal"*, that is, acceptable limit concentrations. If you are reassured by these proclamations then I'm afraid you need a reality check. The studies are often (but not always) based on studies which emanate from the industry itself. The notion that different synthetic chemicals may combine (the cocktail effect) to exhibit toxicity, allergy or chronic disease is missing from the industry perspective. Here, the toxicity (or not) of a given substance is based on assumption, statistical inference and isolated ingestion. Again, the question of why the additives are present in the first place is ignored, circumvented or relegated. If questions were not dismissed in this manner the industry would be open to the detailed scrutiny it so needs to avoid. Aside from these questions the environmental, economic and social impact of *"big agriculture"* is a giant pile of highly visible elephant excreta that will be wholly ignored at FIG and equivalent events.

In a global context, the additives industry is worth hundreds of billions of dollars. There are astronomically huge profits to be made and every section of the industry wants its cut. The machine operates in such a way that it is constantly seeking new creations and applications with which to alter the biochemistry of the food we eat. For example, a portent for the future of bread making in the UK could be the use of a class of proteins known as permeates. [79] These are proteins made from a base of whey protein concentrate, whey protein isolate, ultra-filtered milk, milk protein concentrate and/or milk protein isolate. Now I can take a well educated guess as to what each of these ingredients is, but without looking I couldn't say exactly. By definition, such phrases cannot be seen as clear and informative labelling. Collectively, permeates are supposed to promote the browning of baked goods. They are designed to increase the rate and incidence of Maillard reactions (as discussed in *"the Food Conspiracy book"*). These reactions only occur in the baking oven and give baked foods their characteristic *"browned colour"*. By a stunning coincidence permeates ensure that foods remain softer for longer. The shelf and transportation life will once again be extended. Such possibilities are supposed to elicit an *"oh wow isn't that amazing response"* and for some people, this may well be the case. Yet when the opposite *"so the bread is not really fresh"* or equivalent response occurs great vexation ensues on the part of those who develop novel processing techniques. Now call me Mr. backward if you must but, I would prefer to take a walk to the local high street which is populated by independent butchers, bakers, greengrocers and candle stick makers. I would like to purchase bread that is genuinely fresh and goes stale within a day or so of purchase. I would prefer not see the expertise of food scientists wasted on developing new concoctions and combinations that only exist to serve the vagaries of the food industry. I do not relish the idea of eating food which is laced with additives that the industry is reticent (at best) to discuss. I do not relish the idea of eating food which contains synthetic ingredients whose names I have to look up. I resent, expressing things politely, being seen as the problem for having the audacity to ask or question the motives of a construct which is supposed to exist for my benefit. Finally, are we really going to continue to allow the above kind of practices to continue without any kind of real scrutiny or accountability, I say no, but I am only one of 7 billion (and rising) so it's not really up to me is it?

The span of companies that gather at FIG is not limited to those involved directly in food processing and manufacturing. These huge business concerns see food processing as merely another revenue stream and they act accordingly. The links between the chemical industry and food production are so strong and present that the former is now telling the latter how the food we eat can be altered and increasingly genetically engineered. In the corporate science, I have yet to see one single study or school of thought which asks the *"should"* of such developments. In essence, we are talking about a construct that observes no conflict between manufacturing industrial and agricultural chemicals. The same chemicals that are in processed food are also found in cosmetics, paints, glues and countless other products. A minimum of 6000 and rising different substances are used to adulterate the food we eat. Other estimates put the number at over 10,000 and rising. Some are being replaced or substituted for enzymes and other processing aids. Some additives are clearly necessary but when we look at the ingredients of food X and compare with food A and see that some of the same chemicals are present, questions are bound to be asked. Even more, queries will be raised if it is shown that these same chemicals are manufactured by the chemical and petrochemical industry. The label on a given food product is really the only window we have into the world of food manufacturing. The window itself is made as deliberately opaque as the manufacturers can get away with. If you read the ingredient list on any processed food label it is clear that the substances in question are collated and categorised in such a way that the absolute minimum of information about them is conveyed. As a corollary, if it can be shown that the substance in question is also used in a given manufacturing process, then surely (as a minimum) questions concerning the *"where"*, *"why"* and *"how"* of that substance are more than legitimate. The prevailing assumption from the industry is that *"nature"* does not know best, *"we"* do and *"we"* can make a healthy profit from that supposition too. The true scale of what goes on behind the monolithic and locked down doors of industrial food manufacture truly does beggar belief. The industry can get away with all of this because they have all of this done up like a kipper, locked away in a repository that makes Fort Knox look like a child's piggy bank. This is combined with an extra measure of smoke and mirror slipperiness designed to add to the confusion. These compounds exist to increase the profit margin of the manufacturers. If the sales floor at FIG displays slogans imparting that *"when technology meets nature, you save"* it is difficult to come to any other conclusion. And with that in mind it seems to me that, yes, indeed, it is all about the money and absolutely nothing else.

# Chapter Three: Avoiding Processed Foods

I wrote at the beginning of chapter two that the appraisal of our current catastrophic situation is not a message of doom and gloom, and it isn't, I just don't do denial. Here we are in the 21st century, take a step backward and have a good look at the overall state we are all in. Good isn't it? Just as one set of examples, ask the people of Yemen, Iraq, Syria Northern Nigeria or the Horn of Africa, I'm sure they will be brimming with enthusiasm– that is sarcasm in case you were wondering. Sadly these are not isolated cases or mistakes. They are the consequences of deliberate policy. So, this chapter begins with an easy exercise in personal empowerment. Seriously, take a deep breath and after reading the next section, close your eyes and imagine this scenario. Picture in your mind's eye a world that is run properly. In this world, bad and terrible things do happen but we don't allow what is happening in the Middle East (for example) to potentially drag us all down into the abyss. Nay, we don't allow that particular maelstrom of destruction to fester and grow in the first place. Yet, collectively we have and it is there for all to see, tragically its consequences are not going anywhere any time soon. We have natural disasters; we have crop failures and plenty of conflicts to resolve. The key word here is *"resolved"*, in this imaginary world; our differences are dealt with properly. When a natural disaster happens the destructive impact is dealt with properly. We don't select those places we will help or report on and yes I am talking about Hurricane Harvey, Irma, Liberia, Bangladesh and Northern India as merely the latest examples. People in foreign lands are not left to their own devices (assuming they have any) or supported only by charity. Damage to people, the environment, infrastructure and any property is repaired irrespective of cost as quickly as possible. We do not build new multi-billion aircraft carriers and continually facilitate the means to achieve our own destruction, whilst we cut essential services down to nothing. It is not every person for themselves and tough if you don't make it, or everything you have is destroyed. In this imaginary world, human need and environmental sustainability are of equal importance. Plus, it is realised that you cannot have one without the other and expect to survive. In this world, we have worked together and overcome the instilled, artificial and virulently hateful divisions. These divisions exist for one purpose, which is to distract from the real cause of the horror unfolding all over our once thriving world. Sadly, far too many people here in the UK and abroad have fallen for such divisions hook line and sinker. The whole charade surrounding the UK leaving the EU is but one example of such division. In the desired imaginary world there would be no EU because the historical time lines which led to its inception would never have happened. We would have overcome our differences long ago and would now be working together as one people under one sky under a banner of love, empathy, logic and world peace. People who until very recently were riddled with the sickness of greed, callous disregard, racism and a sense of entitlement that very nearly destroyed our species and the planet which supports all organisms, have woken up and stepped out into the light. For example, in this world:

- There is no need to campaign on processed food because all of our food is grown organically by means of organic and permaculture systems.
- Food processing really means preserving and converting it so that it can be stored and distributed without spoiling.
- There is no need to campaign on GM Food because it doesn't exist.
- There is no need to campaign on climate change because the solutions to it are being implemented at every level of our collective global society. We would not have to be genuinely frightened of those who believe we can control or manage it, or even worse deny its occurrence.
- There is no need to campaign on nuclear issues because

both nuclear weapons and nuclear power have been consigned to a sealed bin labelled *"Warning, Folly Do Not Touch"*. We would not have to worry about the mind set of those who consider either normal or acceptable. They would be in prison or secure hospitals for crimes against life, never mind humanity.

- The profit motive has been subsumed so that services work as services and are beneficial to all in society, not just for the greedy and self-serving elite.
- The mafia and cabal of crooks, thieves, liars, misanthropic, sociopathic and psychopathic criminals who used to run our affairs have been locked up and are receiving the lifelong professional psychiatric help they so desperately need. Or, they are locked up forever in prison where they belong.

I'm sure the reader can add their own individual two pennies worth to this list. Sadly, as things stand it is wholly academic as to what is on the list, for one simple and unfortunate reason. Tragically, we do not live in such a world, not even close. By any benchmark, you wish to choose or by how you would like to cut the cake, we are being dragged into a level of destruction which makes the term mass extinction absolutely appropriate. The tragedy is that we know it is happening, we have the ability, passion, cognisance and individual commitment and means to fix things. There are literally thousands of solutions on the table and some of them are being implemented. Yet globally, nothing like enough is being done, the political will to do what is necessary, is non-existent and we are running out of time. By the time you read this, it will be passed mid- 2017 and I believe by then it will be obvious to all (who choose to look) that on the current trajectory we will be lucky to get through the next couple of decades. Exactly the same thinking applies to avoiding processed foods. The neurosis is obvious. We should not be discussing avoiding any food, processed or otherwise unless you don't like it or can't eat it. We should be celebrating food as part of our collective evolution and culture. The phrase processed food itself should not be a byword for chemically altered gloop that is not fit to be called food and is not by any means good for you. Processed food should represent fresh unaltered food that has been preserved and stored properly thus maintaining its nutritional content. As I have written elsewhere the only reason we are not eating food produced by means of permaculture and/or organic systems is structural. Speaking personally, I have come across frozen processed food that I would not feed to a pet dog, let alone eat myself. However, this is where we are and there are hugely complex systemic issues as to why we are in such a horrible and despiculous (a fusion of the words despicable and ridiculous) position (thanks, Helen!). This chapter will hopefully provide some kind of overview of how we as individuals can avoid processed foods. So here goes.....

The obvious way to avoid processed foods and the additives they contain is to grow your own food and buy the rest from local food retailers and farmers markets. In addition, all the food you prepare and cook ought to be made from scratch with the above fresh and locally sourced ingredients. If you have time and the means to organise in such a way, then you should. The bottom line is clear and precise. When we buy processed food it will almost certainly contain the types of ingredients mentioned and/or discussed in this book. It will also contain staggeringly huge quantities of refined and added salt, sugar and fats. Leaving all other issues aside (for now) if you are purchasing whole foods (even from a supermarket) you are limiting your consumption of such substances. If you are able to purchase your foods from local markets, farmers markets and the like the chances are that you are ingesting even fewer food additives. Sadly, and for *"structural reasons"*, i.e. due to cost, most of us are not in that position. For most of us, any one of these suggestions is going to be difficult to implement so to follow up on all of them is going to be even harder, if not impossible, surely a damning indictment of how our affairs are constructed. From a food perspective, any system which has created a set of circumstances where most of us do not have access to fresh, locally produced *"organic"* food is as flawed as it is dysfunctional. Again and tragically, it is not a question of ability and expertise, how can it be? Human beings have been growing their own food for about 12,000 years. The words *"organic"* and *"superfood"* represent what food is supposed to be like. It is not a status symbol or handy marketing tool; it is food as it is supposed to be. That is tasty, healthy, with texture and absolutely nutritious in the truest sense of the word. Such food is the complete opposite of the processed food we are looking to avoid. The so called food which is the subject of this writing has only really been in existence for the last century and a half or so (see chapter four). Such food is worthy of the term *"processed"* because it has been converted from what was food into something else which is not by definition food. Most of it in comparison to real food is gloop on a plate, it really is. The above statements are not meant to suggest that all additives are bad and that food processing is detrimental to our health and the wider environment. I mean to say, that if we were to be puritanical and preachy about such issues we may as well dispense with the fridge and freezer as well. After all freezing food is a form of food processing as is fermenting blackberries to make wine. The point is to understand what happens in the modern processed food industry, the other related agencies it is connected to and what the objectives of the processing are in the first place. The only reason food is processed in the way it is in the modern age and in the decades running up to it, is to increase profits for the manufacturers, the supermarkets and the economic construct we refer to as *"big agriculture"*. From that perspective, the construct has the additional benefit of concentrating power and control to the detriment of *"how things ought to be done"*.

The cold, hard, and unforgiving reality is that the pace of our lives, the assemblage of our society and the work life balance that we are compelled to endure, makes avoiding processed foods almost impossible. It is crucial to continually reiterate that not all *"additives"* are harmful or unnecessary and that not all *"processed food"* is necessarily bad for you or unhealthy. For example, the packets of chopped vegetables that adorn the supermarket shelves are convenient and not particularly unhealthy. Leaving aside the issues intrinsic to modern agriculture and food distribution, eating a packet mix of fresh frozen vegetables is not from a purely health perspective a bad choice to make. However, if one were to look at how the packet and contents got to your food cupboard and dinner plate, this perspective would have to change. Most processed food does not deliver the nutritional goods, not by a long way too. It also comes with the question *"how did this food get to my dinner plate?"* and all the issues which feed into that question. The words processed and convenience are directly associated with foods which contain a bewildering array of added substances. Many of which the manufacturers are not required to declare. Processing, preserving, pickling and fermenting different foods are not practices unique to the modern world. If we did not employ such techniques then we would not have access to the diversity of food we enjoy. And I would not have fourteen gallons of wine to keep an eye on. However, in the modern world, the majority of processed foods are not healthy or *"good for you"*. With this in mind the sensible reaction if you see that a food is high in fats, sugars, salt and has chemical names (if they are even listed) that you cannot pronounce or just don't make any sense, is to put it back. However, what do you do if you are making a curry from scratch and you want to use fresh ingredients but it's a school night and there is a movie on the TV? Either you get the jar of curry paste and throw it in with the food you are cooking, or you wait until the weekend and make it from scratch. If you are using free range or organic meat, then the cost factor adds a whole new aspect to what should be a simple, rewarding and pleasurable past time. There is a cost in time and money or you end up buying something that contains the ingredients you want to avoid. All I'm saying is that avoiding processed foods is not as easy as it may sound.

For almost all of us avoiding processed foods is going to be nigh on impossible. For example, my nearest local farm shop is four miles away. Most of the food available is fully organically and sustainably certified and boy does it look good, oh yes indeed, it most certainly does. The food and ingredients are of the standard that every person and organism alive on planet Earth should be ingesting. There is also a local farmers market every two weeks on the local high street, which represents a ditto on the quality, taste and appearance of the food on offer. Such outlets sell locally sourced foods which have pretty much come from the farm to the market stall. Often the stall holder will be the person who grew the food and/or reared the animal in question. So you can automatically connect to the producer and avoid the supermarket altogether. In addition, the food miles and proclivity for preservatives, improvers and additives is significantly reduced. It is likely that a local stall in a farmers market will be able to get a regular vegetable box delivery to your household. The vegetables in the box tend to be seasonal. Assuming that you like and can eat the vegetables in the first place two basic choices present themselves. A person can look at that reality and say *"well I don't know what that is so I'm going back to the supermarket"*. Alternatively, you can think *"well I'm going to learn how to cook those vegetables and see what happens"*. Speaking from experience I never really warmed to aubergines or courgettes. So guess what was in one box delivery I got some ten years ago? Yup, you got it, I made a spicy recipe with the aubergine and a herby one with the courgette and you know what it was, surprisingly, more than alright even if I do say so myself. These vegetables are never going to be my favourite but vegetables which come from delivery box schemes do taste nicer and have a richer flavour. The reason is obvious, they are grown properly with the minimum of pesticide and artificial chemicals added. All of this sounds great and I would love to be getting food for our household in this way. Yet again, assuming the option exists, access to such outlets for most of us is denied because it is so much heavier on the wallet. Our household simply cannot afford it, we truly cannot. I surmise hundreds of thousands of households in Britain alone, are in exactly the same position. The **ONLY** reason people do not buy more *"organic food"* boils down to cost. We must remember that *"organic"* and locally sourced food is not free from additives or preservatives. This particular reality taps into the ongoing debate concerning certification of the produce. It also touches on questions concerning whether it is that different from *"non-organic"*, cheaper and more readily available food. However, if you are on a budget it really is an academic question. You are going to buy the best you can afford and sadly for most of us, organic is not going to figure in that particular false choice.

Theoretically, there is plenty more that we as individuals can do. For instance, if you cannot get to an allotment or grow your own vegetables, then you can grow your own herbs. Our household has absolutely no way of doing this either, we have no garden or window boxes. What is more, the local council has bought up all the allotment land and sold it off to property developers. We have the prospect of over 4000 houses being built on green belt land. The development will destroy a thriving, verdant and lush environment and turn it into wholly unnecessary toy town housing. The construction of which could well be well under way by the time you read this book. In a country [1] which has more empty properties than people to fill them, this cannot be a sensible course of action. I would argue that it is absolutely and totally criminal. It will also not be an isolated example; it will be the norm across the UK. We also live literally in the middle of a working farm. So there is no space for us to grow any plants of any description at all. Farm and commercial vehicles, as well as livestock animals, traverse around us on a daily basis. Plus there is no garden or growing space of any kind to call our own. On top of all that, we live in a food desert and that phrase means in our circumstances exactly what it says. Having said all of this, I love where I live and I certainly would not move back to a city.

Another all too common scenario begins to present itself. It makes perfect sense to try and build some sort of financial cushion. You perhaps need this buffer for an unexpected bill, or maybe something has just gone wrong with the family car, or happenstance you have promised the family a holiday somewhere hot later in the year. Irrespective of the specifics for most of us, funds are limited, so if we have to deal with such eventualities or enjoy ourselves, something is going to give. Financial pressure is relieved if you are not eating *"organic"* food regularly. You don't even look because you know you can't afford it. I know our household doesn't, there is no point. Truly, it is that simple and calls to budget, plan and what have you, are not going to change that fact. Personally, one can be forgiven for finding such a position patronising and insulting, well, it gets my back up at any rate. Consider our households own circumstances. There is absolutely no way that we would be able to enjoy the relatively balanced and healthy diet that we have, without the presence of one of the *"discount"* supermarkets. Again, it is that simple. We know how to cook from scratch and nothing is wasted in our household, but without access to relatively cheap and nutritious food, we really would be struggling. If said discount outlet was not here, we certainly would not be eating *"organic",* but we would very much be living off *"beans on toast".* We would need to choose between going to *"alternative music festivals"* or *"eating well"* but we would not be doing both. From a purely financial perspective we cannot complain but please do not be thinking that we are happy with such circumstances because we are not. Underlining the point, the nearest baker we could visit is some three miles away, I have a push bike and exercise is good, so no problem there. However, at a minimum of £2.50 per loaf, it's just not going to happen. This is what living in a food desert means. Your choices are absolutely and totally taken away from you. As far as bread is concerned we have taken to making our own. We are buying organic ingredients and have invested in a bread machine. In the bread department, we have avoided processed food. The food we buy is OK but there is clear room for improvement from every angle you can think of. Most of us have no choice but to frequent the local supermarket. As if that wasn't galling enough, a real gut wrenching kicker is that my meagre amounts of hard earned cash lines the pockets of the very people I despise the most. These people (the suits) represent the ideology that has created our current disgraceful global situation but do not worry or care about its consequences. And every time we go shopping, no matter how unwillingly and with all the awareness we can muster, we are contributing to an ever deteriorating set of global circumstances.

So, how does all of this connect with processed food? For these and other reasons I firmly believe that the best way to avoid processed foods is to stop producing them in the first place. This book is filled with examples of what is meant by *"food processing"*. Hopefully, it will go some way to explaining what has gone so horribly wrong. The examples should also give an indication as to why the current system is not going to last. Getting to grips with avoiding processed food means looking at the entire production and distribution network. At the very least the current system requires a radical overhaul. The profit motive should be driven to the bottom of the priorities list and sustainability catapulted to the top. Referring to the opening section of this chapter, just close your eyes for a minute and really think about what that might mean for every organism on the Earth. We live with the opposite state of affairs. Under capitalism eating processed food in their current wholly unsuitable form is going to continue. The best that we as individuals can do is to avoid them as much as we can where ever we can. The presence of food additives invites controversy, that is, if you are the least bit concerned with what you feed yourself, friends and family with. There are thousands of individual substances collated under the headings listed in

Chapter five. Under such broad strokes are the thousands of substances that are routinely used in modern food processing. The whole area of intensive food production, the processes involved and the chemicals which make it possible is beyond complex. It is overflowing with inter-related arguments, points and counter positions. And despite some removal of E numbers from various own brand food products, the chemicals concerned are absolutely here to stay for the foreseeable future. Such removal is nothing more than an exercise in distraction. The processes themselves do not change merely the chemicals and biological molecules needed to carry them out. Until the entire industry is re-organised, broken up, brought to account for its behaviour and operation and the profit motive subsumed (ideally removed) nothing systemic will change in food manufacturing. If anything the opposite looks set to occur. As with GMO's a school of thought permeates through every level of the industry. As far as the industry is concerned, the science is sound and the testing regime rigorous and so we should not worry about any potential impacts. In this frame, food additives are themselves beneficial and in some cases, they are good for you. The industry position is that additives are not problematic; moreover, their presence ought to be welcomed. Clearly, some additives are absolutely essential and/or nutritionally beneficial. However, the notion that E numbers and GRAS substances are somehow *"good for you"* feeds (pun absolutely intended) into the notion that the industry believes (or projects the position) that it knows better than evolution and nature. Personally, I'm not sure whether to prioritise offence or worry at such a mentality, so I'll give each emotion equal status. Most processed foods contain varying concentrations of synthetic copies or derivatives of the *"natural form"* of a given chemical. Again this is not supposed to be a problem and under the banner of *"substantial equivalence"* (see chapters two and eight) why should it be? Inside this narrative resides a peculiar notion, well to my mind it is more of a justification. The industry wants us to believe eating the copy is not problematic. It does not shy from taking a position whereby it will state that two or more slightly different compounds are the same substance when in reality they are not. One example is the flavour enhancing molecule called mono-sodium glutamate [2] (MSG) or E 621.[3]

## Is Mono-Sodium Glutamate (MSG) Dangerous?

Way back in 1908, or so the story goes, a Japanese Scientist called Kikunae Ikeda [4] was enjoying a bowl of seaweed soup. The soup in question was a mixture of boiled kelp and a fermented stock called Dashi, which is the main ingredient in seaweed called Laminaria Japonica.[5] Dashi gives a whole range of foods an extra savoury flavour. Until 1908 no one knew why, but Ikeda changed all that. In the interests of balance and due credit it is important to highlight that a French Chef called Auguste Escoffier [6] (no, I'm not making the surname up!) was also working in similar territory with European foods. After a year or so of working in the laboratory, Ikeda had managed to isolate the active compound from the L. japonica seaweed. He extracted the dashi from the seaweed as a crystal solid. The chef from France was using veal stock to explore the same taste. In a flagrant breach of laboratory safety standards, Ikeda tasted the crystals he had isolated. From that moment a fifth taste was added to the four (sweet, sour, salty and bitter) already known to exist. According to the literature, Ikeda is reported to have muttered *"delicious"* upon tasting his discovery. Well, if no poetic licence has been granted Ikeda said"oishi" the Japanese word for delicious. Ikeda had discovered glutamic acid ($C_5H_9NO_4$), a non-essential amino acid. The acid is found in varying concentrations in the living organisms which used to live in abundance across the natural world, which itself is enduring systematic destruction. In human beings glutamic acid exists as a substance called glutamate, which has 8 hydrogen atoms. Glutamate is a neurotransmitter [7] whose activity has a direct bearing on our memory, cognisance and learning development. Glutamic acid is the only amino acid manufactured in the brain. Naturally, glutamate exists in foods including hard cheeses [8] (see chapter two), tomatoes, mushrooms, chives and broccoli. By 1909 Ikeda was co-running a company producing glutamic acid. The company was called Ajinomoto, (see chapter 2) or *"essence of taste"* in English. The result of this particular foray into industrial production was the sodium salt of glutamic acid, the substance we know as Mono-Sodium Glutamate (MSG). At the time of writing, Ajinomoto is still the largest producer of MSG on the planet and have their fingers in several pharmaceutical pies to boot as well. In chemistry, a salt is formed when a metal atom takes the place of one or more atoms in a non-metal compound. The formula for MSG is $C_5H_8NO_4Na$, where a sodium atom has replaced one of the hydrogen atoms on the glutamic acid molecule. MSG is well known to induce an *"extra savoury"* or even *"meaty"* taste to the foods it is served with or added to. Since 1909 MSG has been used to induce flavour into just about every food (processed or not) you can think of. The substance is promoted and used as a method to convert the *"bland"* into the *"tasty"*. OK, that is all well and good, but why do the letters MSG have such negative connotations and is it really that dangerous?

The first point to make is the usual sleight of hand employed by the food processors and some of the literature which plays down any dangers (real or imagined) concerning MSG. This book will continually convey that such chicanery is the norm and not the exception. Such sleight of hand is so common that charging the industry with lying and self-serving denial is more than justified. It is absolutely true that glutamic acid and the glutamate compound are present and manufactured naturally by both plants and animals, but these substances are not MSG. Basic chemistry tells us that as soon as you add a different atom to a compound, the proportions of all atoms which make it are changed; we are discussing a different substance. The compounds in question may well be related but they are not the same. MSG was originally made by gently heating seaweed and vegetables in a solution of hydrochloric acid. A compound called acrylonitrile [9] is a precursor substance for the synthetic manufacture of MSG. This method produces mono and di-chloro-propanols which are known carcinogens. [10] As far as cancer is concerned there is no need to panic because most MSG is not produced in this way. However, there is plenty of literature to suggest that food processing and known carcinogens are intertwined with each other. In modern settings, MSG is made by bacterial fermentation of wheat, sugar cane, sugar beet, tapioca or molasses, in the presence of ammonia ($NH_3$). MSG could well be produced by the action of genetically engineered organisms.[11] Tapioca is a starch derived from the cassava plant and sits under the heading modified starch as discussed in chapter two. Molasses are a thick syrupy and dark coloured liquid derived from sugar refining processes. They are a rich source of chemical energy for various fermentation processes and are themselves increasingly likely to be of GM origin. Outside the EU, the source plant matter is likely to be a genetically engineered crop. During fermentation, various species of Corynebacterium [12] use the carbohydrate molecules in the plant matter as a food source. The metabolism of the bacteria produces the glutamate amino acid, which is secreted into a water based (aqueous) solution. The ammonia provides the nitrogen atoms which are necessary for the manufacture of the amino acid. The sodium is added in precise quantities after the fermentation, forming the desired quantities of MSG. Several hundred thousand tonnes of pure MSG are manufactured every year. MSG is one of the most manufactured food additives in the world. MSG works as a flavouring enhancer and is found everywhere in the world of intensive food making. From canned foods to crackers to salads and back again, MSG is likely to be present. It is ubiquitous to Asian cooking; if you have ever seasoned a stir fry the chances are you have used MSG.

As the word implies enhancers intensify certain flavours or tastes which are already present. They do not create new flavours. The intensification occurs when the enhancer interacts by chemical means with substances which are already present in the food. By itself MSG is relatively bland; it is only when it reacts with other substances in the food that the *"umai"* sensation comes forth, which only happens due to the presence of the sodium. It is also why I love marmite with its conjugated *"umami"* or, in English savoury taste so very much. And herein lays the sleight of hand, or flat out lie depending on your degree of militancy. MSG is not glutamic acid, they are different compounds. So when Ikeda and Escoffier (is that a pun I wonder?) both exclaimed *"yum yum"* in their respective languages, it was not due to the presence of MSG, it was due to the presence of glutamate or to be precise a substance called l-glutamate. When animal matter is cooked or when parmesan cheese and tomatoes ripen glutamate breaks down into the l-glutamate form, which gives the food its umami taste. Perhaps this is why homo-erectus became so fascinated with cooking food on the fire. I mean to say imagine how our ancestors must have responded to the difference between raw and cooked food. When animals eat l glutamate the taste receptors are stimulated at the same time. For good reason umami is referred to as the "fifth taste",[13] but umami is not MSG. There is no sodium in l-glutamate or glutamate. Glutamate is 100% made of varying proportions of atoms of hydrogen, carbon, nitrogen and oxygen. In MSG about 21% of the hydrogen is removed and replaced with sodium. Chemically they are not the same molecule and so cannot be considered as the same compound. MSG is not glutamate or l-glutamate and it is here that the rub does reside. MSG and related compounds have been of huge benefit to the processed food industry, the incisive question is to ask *"is MSG dangerous?"*

In 1959 MSG joined a growing list of additives which are in the US Generally Regarded as Safe – for human consumption – or GRAS List (see chapter five) of food additives. It has been there ever since. MSG sits with a continually growing list of substances which may, or may not be fit to reside under the GRAS heading. By 1969 a condition known as Chinese Restaurant Syndrome [14] (CRS) had become recognised by the *"medical literature"*. Today, the same condition is known as MSG system complex. It means that excessive consumption of MSG can cause symptoms ranging from asthma and shortness of breath, to palpitations and nausea to head aches and fatigue. Longer term consumption has been linked to obesity, glaucoma and even depression. Chapter six discusses the term excito-toxin as applied to that other much-maligned food additive aspartame. An excito-toxin is any substance (normally an amino acid) which over stimulates the cells of the nervous system. The cells become over worked and in sensitive individuals the extra stimulus can intensify or bring on learning difficulties, Huntingdon's chorea, Alzheimer's and Parkinson's disease as well as a syndrome called Lou Gehrig's disease [15] (ALS). This can happen because when it is metabolised the glutamate portion of the MSG molecule interacts with any glutamate receptors in the body. These receptors can be in the heart, the pancreas or the brain in fact, anywhere in the body that glutamate is needed. It is needed in many places and so has many functions in both plants and animals, glutamate is everywhere in the natural world. For instance, the heart functions to pump blood and every substance dissolved in it around the body. One of the mechanisms which enable the heart to function as it should is the cardiac cycle. [16] Naturally produced glutamate molecules (i.e. those made by your metabolism) regulate the cardiac cycle by keeping the electrical conductivity of the heart within precise and narrow homeostatic limits. The heart is beating in balance with the other metabolic processes going on in the body. Too much glutamate irrespective of the source will disrupt (amongst other mechanisms) the cardiac cycle. The result is cardiac arrhythmias, to you and I that means heart palpitations of varying severity. Science understands that should levels of magnesium drop, the sensitivity of the glutamate receptors is known to increase. The same is true of other trace metals too. Consequently, negative health impacts of varying intensity are much more likely for a given input of glutamate molecules. None of this is to suggest that MSG will definitely cause harm; indeed plenty of people consume moderate amounts with no impact on their health. However, the point remains, if you are sensitive to MSG or its metabolites you could well exhibit some form of intolerance. Writing personally, I find the position that concerns *"do not stand up to scientific scrutiny"* [17] patronising, superior and dismissive. It is spurious to equate the presence of natural forms of ingredients in fresh food with artificial variants in processed food. Stating that the two are identical, and then combining them in the diet, then marking them as equivalent is problematic to a point at or close to criminality. The substantial equivalence position also conveniently ignores the three questions which thread throughout this writing.

Natural substances have evolved to be where they are for a reason. We ought not to be using the existence of an evolved substance as a reason to justify adding a synthetic variant, (which is not the same molecule), into the human food chain. I find the attitude that people do not need to be told what they are eating because there is no scientific [18] basis for doing so, to be shocking but not surprising in its excessive scientific arrogance. It is similar to the attitude concerning GMO's and the scientific case thereof. If you are framing your support or opposition to a given activity, substance, process, or decisions of any kind, then you need to realise that the scientific case is only one component of a larger argument. As with GMO's the supporters absolutely dismiss with that *"you must be from Mars look"* when you start to ask questions like, *"well why does this substance exist in the first place and who is really benefitting from its presence"?* As with aspartame, the manufacturers have to state that a given product contains MSG. However, by a clean label sleight of hand (see chapter 2) they do not have to say which foods contain free glutamic acid, even though it is the base molecule for MSG. Even though you may be avoiding some MSG the chances are that you are not avoiding extra inputs of glutamic acid. If a food is processed it is likely to contain MSG or similar glutamate based molecules. The only way to genuinely avoid eating it is to not eat processed food, which is all well and good if you can. Yet to avoid ingesting MSG completely the best way would be not to manufacture it at all. Failing that, don't we have the right to decide whether to add it the food we eat? Perhaps, at the very least give people a choice as to whether they want it on their food or not. As an absolute minimum, perhaps MSG should not be added to food at all. Perhaps it should be sold in a similar way to salt and pepper. Perhaps if food was produced with the intention of providing healthy and nutritious food for everyone on the planet, if trust had not been so brutally violated then perhaps controversies, (real or imagined) concerning MSG and other substances would not exist. Against that backdrop lays the distressing reality of over a billion people wondering where their next meal is coming from. Controversies and questions do exist and with good reason too!

## Artificial Sweeteners

Chapter six discusses in some detail the very real issues and concerns with artificial sweeteners that those who ingest them really ought to have. This section of text was initially the concluding section of that chapter. In the interest of balancing up this writing, I put this section here. So as the signposting point made in the introduction makes clear a good direction for the reader to take after this chapter, even after this section would be chapter six. Before carrying out the research for this book I had no idea about the chemistry, biochemistry and metabolism of artificial sweeteners. If I'm honest I didn't think they were potentially harmful or dangerous. I was only concerned about the regulatory framework and construct which allowed the approval of additives in general and sweeteners in particular. I certainly had no real idea of the potential harm that the entire family of compounds could cause in human populations. Now, I firmly believe that there is no such thing as a completely safe artificial sweetener. We are only just beginning to understand the very real biological consequences of consuming the whole plethora of additives, processing aids, preservatives and indeed artificial sweeteners. We have no real idea of the long term consequences of excessive artificial sweetener consumption. We have no idea of the long term consequences for the brain or our metabolism of continually ingesting substances which trick the brain into thinking it is receiving an energy source which does not exist. Going further, I believe there to be a case for a complete and total ban on their manufacture. As a believer in the precautionary principle, the answer is obvious. Artificial sweeteners appear to be making the health of the populations that ingest them worse than it would be if they were not available. Chapter six presents the case that they are wholly unnecessary and only exist to satisfy a manufactured demand for a wholly synthetic family of chemicals. These substances have no business being in existence in the first place. They certainly ought not to be routinely added to food, drink and medicines. Globally, the quantities we are speaking of are huge and the sweetener industry itself is worth hundreds of millions of dollars. It is becoming clear that artificial sweeteners are contributing to the burgeoning global obesity epidemic. The therapies used to treat it represent a revenue stream into the already bloated pockets of big pharma. In that frame surely one method to guarantee that they won't contribute to ill health and add to obscene levels of profit, is to stop making them, here in the UK and abroad. All existing sweeteners have some potential to induce metabolic harm and the next generation have at least equal potential. Failing an outright ban, which is not going to happen any time soon, a good strategy would be to adopt your own precautionary approach and avoid them completely. As for sugar, well, the ethical, moral, economic and environmental and health concerns around it are just as clear and present as those intertwined with artificial sweeteners. The only saving grace for sucrose is that it is a natural and plant sourced sweetener. If you are reading this book in the UK, the sugar you buy is likely to be from a domestic source. Arguably, it has less of an environmental impact than sugar produced in other parts of the world. The human body can cope with sugar even if it is refined much more readily than the sweeteners. Aside from that concerns about sugar neatly dovetail into those of sweeteners. I would advocate avoiding added sugar where ever possible. We have recently taken to using unrefined natural and organic sugars of one form or another. As far as coffee is concerned a friend mentioned maple syrup, which we now enjoy instead of sugar. Sadly, the only certifiable real deal and organic brand we could find and afford is imported from Canada in a plastic bottle. The bottle is sturdy and will be put to another use, but that is not the point is it? We hope that enough maple trees are grown to offset the carbon emissions. It goes on and on and well and truly you cannot win! Coffee and tea themselves present a whole host of equivalent issues which means that when our household can afford it we buy fair trade and/or organic brands whenever we can. This does nothing about the prolific use of water to grow these cash crops. It also taps into the question of "*why is so much arable land in far off countries is set aside to feed the caffeine addiction of the industrialised world*"? To be clear, caffeine is the most consumed stimulant in the world and by a long way too. Aside from all of that, the only refined sugar I knowingly ingest comes from processed food. So we avoid that as much as we can too. It is for the reasons presented in this chapter (and others which are not) that I choose not ingest artificial sweeteners. It is a contradiction to say that I use refined sugar to sweeten the coffee and tea I drink and in the fruit wine I make. On the last point, we have decided to go for organic white sugar. Again it's the cost of "*organic*" sugar, it is between twice and three times the price of the supermarket brand we used to buy. Plus, it will likely have to be delivered if we are to avoid passing any of our hard earned to the supermarkets. Truly when you start to try and take control you wonder what the point is. However, by doing so I have made the issues presented in this chapter a personal irrelevance. As such artificial sweeteners reside under the banner *"stupid choices"* mentioned in chapter four. Having said all of that we are going to keep exploring other options in the sweet stakes, instead of reaching for hot liquids which contain suspended caffeine carrying particles I will be going for water and fresh fruit where ever I can. We then reach into questions about where the fruit comes from, how it is made, who grew it, how it is transported. Or more incisively I ask *"where does my hard earned travel as it goes back through the resource chain from retailer to initial producer"?* Ad infinitum stupid choices do indeed continually present themselves.

## Food is made from the elements of life.

Here is a startling fact for you to digest; yes that pun is intended, so here goes. All the food we eat and all the molecules which compose our bodies and that of every organism on Earth are made of the atoms of the same six elements. The elements in question are Carbon, Hydrogen, Nitrogen, Oxygen, Phosphorous and Sulphur, or "The CHNOPS" [19] for short. Trace metals are bonded into the molecules made from these six atoms, but every organism on Earth is held together by the chemistry of these non-metal elements. Plenty of healthy foods contain trace amounts of known toxins. For instance:

- Apple seeds contain trace amounts of cyanide and similar compounds
- Cabbage, spinach, strawberries, soybeans, pears, peaches, cauliflower, kale and broccoli can be goitrogenic [20] if consumed in large amounts.
- Mustard oils can increase cholesterol levels and/or cause the growth of fat cells in and around the heart.
- Citrus fruits, carrots and parsnip can induce hypersensitivity to UV radiation, thus increasing the risk of skin cancer.

- Kidney beans, wheat and rye can interfere with the uptake, absorption and break down of carbohydrates.
- Lectins which are found in pulses can prevent the absorption of essential nutrients from partially digested food in the stomach.

The list is, endless, yet nobody is saying avoid these foods, quite the opposite. And speaking personally I chow down on these and other staple foods pretty much every day. However, it is at best spurious to

Equate the presence of natural substances, toxic or otherwise, with the cocktail of additives which call the western diet home. The notion that we have evolved over thousands of years to accommodate the presence of naturally occurring substances is entirely missing from the establishment position. The vast majority of the substances discussed in this book are synthetic copies of the natural form. Most of which we have not evolved to metabolise in isolation from the organism they came from. Clearly, this applies to the compounds added to the processed foods we are seeking to avoid. This is part of the reason why so many people report negative food and related issues. The industry, its apologists and appeasers are at best reticent to discuss such viewpoints. Perhaps it is too close to their comfort to look in the mirror.

The food industry cannot escape the fact that every product churned out from its factories is made from the elements and compounds which are hardwired into the fabric of life itself. It is very keen for all of us to believe that synthetic copies are the same as the natural form. The synthetic form is a direct and exact chemical copy of the natural form. The same atoms are present, they are bonded to each other in the same way and they exist in the same proportions. As far as the industry is concerned both forms are identical. Processed food is crammed to the hilt with refined sugars, salt and various fats, none of which have a designated e number. These substances along with colourants, additives, flavour enhancers and the like exist to disguise the real appearance and taste of the slurry that comes from the waste exhaust pipe of the entire processed food industry. For the manufacturers, the synthetic substances are not responsible for any reported negative health problems. These substances are needed to make processed food appealing to the population. A point no agency or individual which has a vested interest in the construct itself is ever going to admit, well not publicly at any rate. And the industry will say and do anything it can to maintain this position. For example, take a look at the developing hoo hah around the *"sugar tax"* on carbonated soft drinks. The usual suspects have bought the law and turned the whole issue into a giant global farce. Profits will be maintained at the health expense of those who continue to buy soft fizzy drinks. Still, money has been made and interests have been protected, so no problem hey? Personally, I find such inhumanity, simplistic justification, denial of reality and abrogation of responsibility offensive to a point well-passed criminality. If we want to really deal with the intensifying and expanding (pun intended) global obesity epidemic, then changing the way the foods responsible are made would be a good start. Artificial sweeteners and High Fructose Corn Syrup (see chapter seven) could be removed out right, thus dealing with any health related issues immediately. It is not possible to separate food processing and additives; they are inextricably linked with each other. Many nutritionists and clinical dieticians believe and publicly state on the basis of sound, objective and value free science that additives are not problematic and even that they are good for you. This perspective maintains that all additives are subject to rigorous testing, are regulated and will be withdrawn if necessary. In this frame, there can be no problem with their unrestrained use. Fresh foods do contain the type of natural toxins and other substances mentioned above. The industry is not shy about imparting that their products can be better for you because they have removed such substances from the food in question. Here, processed food is healthier than the unadulterated, unprocessed *"straight out of the ground"* and fresh food that we are supposed to be eating. Clearly, this writer disagrees in the strongest possible terms and this writing is a plea for you the reader to take the same position. To reiterate a recurrent theme, the above position ignores the reality that the only reason people (including yours truly) buy what is on offer is because most of us have no choice, but to do so.

In a related arena, the biotechnology and life science industries continually undermine any point of view which contradicts its own assertions concerning GMO's. Those who see no issue with food additives in general and E numbers in particular because they have been scientifically tested, really need to think outside the scientific box. The essential point is to ignore the science concerning the safety or not of a given additive, e number or processing aid. I mean to say:

- *"So what?"* if the UK Food Standards Agency (FSA) or its European equivalent the European Food Safety Authority (EFSA) states that substance X is safe.
- *"So what?"* if the US FDA and other regulatory authorities tell us that GMO's are safe or *"substantially equivalent"* to non-GM varieties.
- *"So what?"* if a chemical is on the GRAS list.
- *"So what?"* if a representative of the industry says substance X is perfectly safe.

Why do I say *"so what"*? Well, I don't trust you because of what you represent. I don't want your food and I'm not eating it, as much as I can't. As best I can I absolutely reject your position in any way that I can, until I have reason to think and act differently. The point is to question the process, application or technique being employed in the first place. From that position, you can start to look at the alternatives (that is organic and permaculture systems) which already exist. Growing food and rearing animals properly has proven benefits which far outstrip the bare faced lies emanating from the food industry, the supermarket chains and the construct we refer to as *"big agriculture"* [21]. Similarly, there is an equally entrenched point of view which holds that because food allergies are often caused by the chemicals contained in natural foods, the additives or processing techniques cannot be at fault. And so it goes on.

The science practised by the food industry is worlds apart from the corpus of knowledge I value and respect with every fibre of my being. Science in all its forms exists as a mechanism to make sense of the world and universe around us. It should serve all of humanity and not be used to line the pockets of a privileged few at our expense. Science is not infallible, it is a human construct and it errs in just the same way as you or I do. In a food context chapter five shows how substances that were once thought safe were used with no regulation or regard for any consequences. In the modern world, there are plenty of nutritionists, dietitians, food scientists and health care professionals who do not agree that additives are *"good for you"*. From that perspective, the bottom line is that fresh, unprocessed or natural foods are a much better nutritional bet. At this juncture, it seems pertinent to ask the reader, if they had to choose between the two positions, *"who would you believe and why"?* I would add that if you as an individual have no problem with eating food which contains unnecessary additives, then please do carry on. However, that is up to you, so, don't tell me or anyone else that I/we should do the same, and please do take *"that"* look off of your face. It is your choice and not mine or anyone else's. I and the hundreds of millions of people here in the UK and abroad continue to move in the opposite direction. The above position (along with the assertions of those who support GM crops) ignores the human rights dimension to the argument. I choose to avoid processed food where ever possible. A quick perusal of the price of *"healthy"* and *"organic"* food demonstrates in the strongest possible terms that most of us are unable to make a *"fair choice"*. We simply cannot afford the extra outlay and so we do what we can, where ever we can. Carrying on, irrespective of subjective opinions around taste and texture, I would choose to avoid any food which I knew to contain GMO's or was laden with additives if a plate of real food was in the offing. On top of all that, I would rather eat a plate of food sourced from producers in my locale. I would impart that all things being equal *"isn't that my right and yours?"* Any person, organisation or agency that tells you different has the problem and not you the reader. It never fails to stagger me that when one looks at the price differential between *"processed"* and *"unprocessed"* food, the former is invariably less expensive than the latter. As the portion of *"natural"* substances in a given food increases so does the price. This reality is discussed with real examples in chapter four. I would ask those who ignore or accept such points *"how in the name of common sense and basic humanity can that be right?"* You should not need to read primary scientific literature to come to the appropriate conclusion, i.e. it isn't right. If you need an explanation on this point, then in the strongest possible terms I argue that you have no business in telling me or anyone else what is good to eat and what is not. At this juncture, it is again crucially important to state that some additives are beneficial and necessary. Many substances delimited by an E number have been with us for millennia. Plus, additives per se are not the preserve (Ha! There goes another intentional pun), of intensively produced food. They are everywhere and there are plenty of additives in organic and artesian foods.

Aside from other dietary time bombs, the modern world is enduring an obesity epidemic which is largely of its own making. The food manufacturers produce food which is directly linked to obesity and its bedfellow type-2 diabetes (T2D). It is allowed to operate because the global political establishment benefits financially and materially from the production and consumption of the food too. Neither agency has any real interest in stopping it. If they did the food would not be made. I am not in favour of *"sugar tax"* on fizzy drinks. I do not believe such strategies will get to the root of the problem, the manufacture of the products themselves. Any revenue raised will only be recycled into the economy, in much the same way as the revenue raised from taxing tobacco and petrol is. In this context we can further ask:

- Is it really so outlandish to suggest the existence of strong and real connections between the consumption of processed food and the incidence of *"negative food issues"* reported by millions of individuals?
- Is it really so outlandish to suggest that a large part of the blame for the steady increase in the incidence of chronic disease can be laid at the door of intensive food making?

I don't think so. It is not as clear cut as this and there are other factors at work here. All I am imparting is that if *"the diet"* can be improved and if the manufacture of *"unnecessary processed food"* is discontinued, then likely we would see an almost immediate drop in T2D and obesity. This is not rocket science or quantum mechanics; there are several strands of thought which give these questions credence. If it is true that two-thirds of the UK population is overweight and about a quarter of that number are clinically obese then grounds for concern must present themselves. Clearly, there are questions of personal responsibility and education intertwined with all of this. However, if a community does not have outlets for fresh fruit and vegetables then from a nutritional perspective things are scuppered before they have even begun. Speaking personally, I have been on the *"campaign trail"* and been *"on the knocker"* talking with people in locations which only have a takeaway, a corner shop and a small under stocked supermarket as the only food options available. Unless a household has transport or access to it, fresh food in many communities might as well only be available on Alpha Centauri. Little wonder, that the health of the nation appears to be suffering the consequences of the lack of availability of fresh, wholesome, locally sourced and/or grown fruit and vegetables and other foods to boot! In areas where such food is not available or indeed affordable nutrition and health are abstract concepts which have no bearing on the daily lives of the people who live there.

I am not a culinary saint I have eaten my share of ready meals, takeaways and all the forms of junk food that you can think of. For example, back in the day, I used to enjoy a pot noodle and dunk crisps into it too. And yes I do hark back to those Halcyon care free days, but not very often! And you know what; if *"I'm on the go"* the chances are that I will eat the sort of food made by the construct I have eviscerated here. If you pick up any food in a jar, packet or freezer in your local supermarket it is going to contain some of the many thousands of food additives that exist in the human food chain. However, you only have to read the ingredient list of any processed food product to realise that additives are omnipresent and so are almost impossible to avoid. Once you start to dig a little (and over the last two years I've certainly done plenty of that) you really do begin to realise just how intertwined the relationship between *"food processing"* and the product you are buying really is. The food and related industries operate under a veil of secrecy that puts the machinations of Stalinist Russia to shame. Over the last few decades, the opacity has been maintained under meaningless euphemisms designed to divert, obviate, obfuscate as well as overwhelm and confuse all those who inquire as to what is really going on behind the industry closed doors. Finding out what is in the food you eat, where it came from, why it is there and how it is produced is a journey into a world of smoke and mirrors that demotivates all but the most determined individuals and/or campaigning organisations. Since the 1990's the manufacturers have sought to protect their activities under the banner of confidentiality, deregulation, competition and protecting intellectual property. The actions of successive governments have not helped matters either. For instance, in 1996 the dying putridness of John Major's conservative government allowed the use of enzymes in food processing to become a free for all with no accountability or scrutiny. More succinctly in 1996, the use of enzymes in food processing was completely deregulated. Sadly, the loathsome Tony *"bomber"* Blair and the poisonous new labour project kept things going and that included GMO's. Today it is almost impossible to contact the manufacturers directly; any queries are now dealt with by the retail outlets, i.e. the supermarkets. The cold harsh truth is that most of us know very little about the food on the supermarket shelves. Try this simple experiment:

- Go to your *"larder"* and pick any processed food product and check how many individual ingredients or classes of ingredients there are.
- Then ask yourself *"do I know what that means?"* I'm willing to bet (and I don't gamble) that the list of those you know is going to be short.
- Then, have a look at the ingredients and find out what you can about them.
- Then ask yourself *"do I really want to be eating that?"* Again as a non-gambler, I'm willing to bet that the answer is *"no"* for most of what you find.
- Then pick the food with the most ingredients and additives that you don't know about and then contact the shop that you bought it from.
- Ask to speak with someone involved in purchasing, a person who makes decisions about what products to buy. Do not be lambasting the check-out staff or the owner of your local corner shop.
- Then see what happens and what kind of response you get.
- Then ask yourself if any response you get makes any sense.
- Finally, ask yourself do you believe the response.

Try this several times and I'm pretty sure that you will find that avoiding processed food is not as easy as it sounds. As I am very fond of saying during discussions on complex issues, *"things are just not that simple"*. As individuals we can all *"do our bit"*, we can all learn to cook and we can all get the best ingredients we can afford. However, the huge elephant poo in the middle of the room is the manufacture of the food itself. While it still exists, genuinely avoiding the western diet and the processed food which composes most of it is all but impossible. This Book will hopefully keep reiterating that the sooner the manufacturing stops and the poo is removed, a better place our world will be.

# Chapter Four: Examples of chemical gloop, disguised as food, we used to eat

The next time you go shopping take a look at the ingredients list of the processed food you buy. I have tried it more than several times over the last few years. Without pushing it I would also suggest that if you treat your children with *"pester items"* that you do the same with those as well. At the very least it would be good to know what you are feeding them, wouldn't it? For all the wrong reasons looking at the ingredients is a truly eye opening experience, or it should be! It also goes some way to explaining the general tone of this book. Without exception I have looked at the ingredients list and thought either *"what is that?"* or *"why is it there?"* or both! It is very simple, most of these substances should not be present in the food we eat. Indeed a healthy percentage should not exist at all. A quick look at the ingredients list on processed food indicates the realities of 21st century food processing. Wherever possible the manufacturers have substituted the *"natural"* for the *"artificial"*. And have converted the healthy and wholesome, into the exact opposite as they have done so. Having said that, the industry does seem to be getting the message that we as *"the public"* are increasing our awareness [1] of what is in the food we eat. However, as chapter two discusses I do not expect the industry to make any real changes any time soon. I do predict another major case of food related *"label and ingredient wash"* now and in the very near future. The recent shenanigans in mid-2017 concerning the size of chocolate [2] bars, pizzas and ready meals here in the UK is a developing clear cut example. One factor is absolutely clear, the size or portions of these packaged foods may well come down, but their price won't. Based on such movements I fully expect a fresh set of artificial sweeteners (see chapter seven) to take the place of the refined sugar in confectionery. This will likely create a whole new set of food related problems which the industry will ignore and/or project the responsibility for on to the population. In a capitalist world, the only reason such changes happen is to increase profits. By 2017 we now have a criminally ludicrous situation whereby profits are increased in direct proportion to the quantities of additives used. The industry has bought or watered down the law to such an extent, that it is normal to label a given food as *"XYZ"* even when it does not contain any of the *"natural"* substances one would think it would contain, based on what is stated on the label. The construct is able to advertise its products as something which they are not. When raw foods are processed by industrial means, they are:

- Heated
- Extracted
- Hydrogenated
- Genetically modified
- Chemically modified
- Nutrified (see chapter one and below) with synthetic copies of essential nutrients
- Treated with synthetic and chemical preservatives
- Dehydrated

The Western diet is characterised by food which is converted from that which *"came out of the ground"* into a form where the only similarity processed food has to unprocessed food is the name. The vitamins and minerals have been removed and are then replaced in precise quantities, often less than those originally present. The replacements are often synthetic variants of those originally present. Replacing nutrients which have been lost during the processing regime is called enrichment. Fortification is concerned with adding nutrients to food which were not originally present. Together both terms are known as nutrification. An example of fortification would be the addition of iodine to salt (to prevent goitre [3]) or the addition of vitamin D to milk (to prevent rickets [4]). Powdered milk also contains added quantities of vitamin A and D. Examples of enrichment would include the addition of iron and B vitamins to processed flour or the addition of folic acid to breakfast cereals. Once again the reasons as to why both practices are so necessary in modern food processing are not a subject the industry is keen to discuss. Thousands of individual foods have been enriched or fortified and the total number is rising steadily. To my mind, both practices would be unnecessary if we all had access to healthy, nutritious and affordable food as the basis for a genuinely balanced diet. There is no sensible reason as to why this is not the case. As chapter three makes abundantly clear, the only reason why people buy processed food is a disordered fusion between low affordability and low availability. In very broad strokes the only reason most nutrification happens is due to the food processing regimes themselves. Aside from *"medical reasons"* or *"specific circumstances"* I see no sensible reason for such practices. If the *"food system"* were organised differently, neither enrichment nor fortification would be necessary on anything like the scale that it occurs. The health of humanity could be revolutionised in a few short years, say a decade at worst. As individuals, we would not need to make the kind of stupid choices outlined below. Why? The food most of us are compelled to eat would not exist; we would be eating food as it should be eaten as it has evolved to be eaten.

## Selection One: Blackcurrant Cordial

During the course of our lives, most of us have drunk fruit squashes and cordials. This first example concerns the ingredient list in the black currant juice that we used to buy. To be fair underneath the large letters which say *"Black Currant Juice"* smaller letters declare *"flavour cordial"*. Above the ingredient list, we have a declaration of *"concentrated black currant flavour soft drink with sugar and sweeteners"*. So, I guess the manufacturer is not being completely spurious or misleading. However, I would feel better if the liquid was not labelled as a juice because it isn't. A juice is a liquid that you collect when you press a fruit or vegetable. To be considered pure and fresh nothing must be added and nothing must be taken away. (See choice 3 below). These are the substances listed in order, in the flavour cordial concoction:

- Water, yes water $H_2O$ complete with dipole moment and everything!
- Citric Acid (E 330 [5])
- Colours (caramel E 150d [6])
- Anthocyanins: A hugely important class of flavonoid [7]compounds, which belong to the phenol family of organic molecules (see chapter one). The Flavonoids are discussed in the *"medicine on your plate"* series of books.
- Acidity regulator (sodium citrate): E 331 [8] these compounds are found in organisms across the natural world. It is almost certain that the regulator in this drink will not be a natural form.
- Flavourings: Tellingly, no specific chemicals are listed.
- Preservatives: Sodium Benzoate (E 210 [9]) and Potassium Sorbate (E 202 [10]).
- Sweeteners: Aspartame (see chapter six) and Sodium Saccharin (E 954 [11]). The latter compound is the sodium salt [12] of saccharin, itself the oldest sweetener on the planet. Both forms of saccharine are discussed in chapter seven.

If you look at the ingredients on most squashes and cordials, you will notice that water is at the top of the list. For most of these drinks water is the main ingredient and the same is true of most carbonated fizzy drinks. The other substances are dissolved in the water and the chances are that any real fruit juice comes from a concentrate. [13] Another glaringly apparent point to make is so obvious that it hurts! It is the same point that will run throughout the examples mentioned in this chapter. Yup, you got it; there is no black currant juice or even concentrate in this cordial. I've had a look at other brands too, and most squashes do not contain the juice of any fruit whatsoever. Some are better than others, but very few contain the fruit juice they are supposed to be made from. Take a look at the ingredient list in any cordial you may have and see for yourself. The purple liquid under discussion here is not an isolated example (see chapter four). Other types of cordial also contain anything but the juice from the fruit in question. These are the realities of cheaper or *"bottom of the range"* brands of cordial. The reader should not be surprised when I write that as the juice percentage increases so does the price. Organic and health food brands are the most expensive cordials available. We buy one litre as needed from the local health food shop. Sometimes this is not possible, so we buy a brand from the local supermarket, which contains (so it says) 50% real fruit juice, this may or may not be true. However, it doesn't really matter, because it contains aspartame (see chapter six), an artificial sweetener that really ought to be banned, but not for the reasons you may be thinking. Why not buy another brand? Is the obvious, almost knee jerk response. Well, because they all contain aspartame and other sweeteners but much less (if any) real fruit juice, than the 50% fruit juice brand. Such are the trade-offs one has to make in a consumer society! Such simple realities also thread into the position taken in Chapter 3. If we are serious about avoiding processed food, then how it is manufactured has to be, as a minimum, radically overhauled. Food manufacturing must be converted to a mechanism that provides healthy, wholesome food for the entire population of this planet. At the moment it does the exact opposite.

## Selection Two: Ice Cream

Modern food production is characterised by the routine and prolific substitution of existing substances with others that would not be there if the food was not processed. A common example of this practice occurs in the manufacture of ice cream. Have a look at this ingredient list and see if you can spot the flaw:

- Reconstituted skimmed milk
- Water
- Milk sugar
- Glucose/dextrose syrup
- Coconut milk
- Milk Proteins
- Palm oil
- Emulsifiers: Mono and di glycerides of fatty acids (E 471 – 479b [14])
- Stabilisers: Guar gum (E 412 [15]) and sodium [16] alginate [17] (E 401 [18])
- Flavourings: Vanilla beans
- Colour: Annatto (E 160B [19])

Did you spot the flaw? Yes, that's right; there is no cream, at all, anywhere in the product. What we had inadvertently bought is a dessert which uses water and additives held together in a solid cohesive structure in the freezer. As long as the dessert can remain solid for long enough outside of the freezer we can enjoy according to the manufacturers *"smooth vanilla, velvety ice – cream with delicious real vanilla"*. Except that when we found out it has no cream and that it is unlikely to contain any real vanilla, such proclamations are meaningless. Nothing else is real in this fake ice cream so why should the vanilla be? By any objective standard, they are flat out lies. Since discovering this particular reality, we have not bought any ice cream which is not ice cream. For budgetary reasons and because I have no sweet tooth, ice cream is now in a box labelled *"special treat"*. It shouldn't be but it is. The only reason we did not bin the above mixture straight away comes down to the belief that it is immoral to throw food away, even if it does not match what is written on the label. The plastic container is somewhere in the wine fruit freezer, filled with fruit. It will once again be put to good use when the picking season comes around again. So what of the ingredients in the yellow gloop labelled as ice cream? I have what you might call something of a scientific background. In addition to my continuing research on the issues mentioned at the beginning of chapter two, I have also spent the last few years looking into food and food related issues. I have some idea as to what the terms in the above and other ingredient lists mean. Without sounding conceited, insulting, superior or patronising, even with that background I still had to look most of these ingredients up. Something I have been doing lots of over the last couple of years. A habit I strongly advise you to take up. For example, sodium alginate is extracted from seaweed and is an essential ingredient in the antacid formulation we in the UK call Gaviscon. The emulsifiers are also found wherever the industry needs to integrate them into its practices. The bread discussed in *"The Food Conspiracy Book"*, is but one example. The same is true of the palm oil which is present to give the misnamed ice cream its structure. The term *"reconstituted"* is just another word for rehydration of powdered milk. The original milk has been dried out and converted to powder. Then a precise amount of water is added to it to make a given processed food, in this example non-ice cream.

Natural annatto [20] has been employed as a food colouring or pigment agent for centuries. It induces a deep reddening effect and so has also been used as a dye for hundreds of years. Annatto comes from the seeds of the achiote plant which is native to the tropical regions of Latin and Central America. The active ingredient is a carotenoid substance called bixin [21]. The seeds themselves are about 5% pigment but over three-quarters of that figure is bixin. Annatto is known to reduce blood pressure and kill bacteria. It is also known to be effective in treating minor burns and wounds as well as with the prevention of some visual impairments. The seeds are also a rich source of tocotrienols [22] which are chemically similar to vitamin E. The tocotrienols and related compounds are believed to prevent the liver from producing the Low-Density Lipo-protein (LDLP [23]) form of cholesterol. The bad stuff that you don't want in your veins and arteries! Annatto is denoted by the number E 160b [24]. As a colourant, it has largely replaced tartrazine [25] (E 102), which is one of the *Southampton 6* [26] compounds. These compounds and sodium benzoate have been implicated in contributing to hyperactive behaviour in children. The Southampton six story is but one of a series of controversies [27] which represent a running sore. I write of a pustule that has percolated throughout the recent history of UK food law, public health, as well as notions of trust in science. However, this is another deeply complex and interconnected story that I just cannot do the justice it so richly deserves here in this book. So I'm afraid you'll just have to wait and watch this space. So, let's get back to our non-ice cream. Annatto is often used in tandem with curcumin (E 100 [28]) which is derived from the turmeric plant. Curcumin acts as both a colourant and preservative. It can be extracted by traditional methods from the parent plant. There are no known toxic effects of consuming dietary levels of curcumin. Yet, all substances have the ability to elicit undesired effects and curcumin is no different. Curcumin promotes the release of bile in the liver, and so aids with digestion. As with annatto, it is often extracted by chemical means. Almost certainly it will be synthetic forms that are used by the manufacturers. Similarly, (at time of writing) there are no known toxic consequences of ingesting annatto. However, the seeds contain a wide range of active chemicals and can induce allergic reactions (which most substances can); in extreme cases, it can elicit anaphylactic shock. It has been known to provoke IBS [29] in some individuals, but to date, there is no causative link between annatto and the syndrome. More pressingly, people with diabetes or those about to go to surgery are generally advised to limit and monitor their intake. Annatto can increase blood sugar levels. In traditional circumstances, annatto seeds are soaked in water and oil, gently heated so that the active part of the seed is separated out. The resulting oil based paste can then be used directly in cooking, or it can be dried and stored. Clearly, this does not happen in the magnificent world of food processing. The seeds are gently heated to about 70°C and then agitated in vats containing food grade vegetable oil. The mixture is concentrated such that it contains about 8% bixin and other pigments. However, the manufacturers are looking to replace the oil with propylene glycol [30]. By the time this book is published, it may have happened. This is a wholly synthetic compound derived from the refining of crude oil. It has dozens of uses and applications ranging from antifreeze to cosmetics. It is also on the GRAS [31] list discussed in chapter five and has been used in medicine for the last half century. So why is a swap being planned? Well, the official reason is that the glycol is more effective at extracting the active ingredients from the seeds. And that may well be true for the annatto and other substances present in the seeds; however, the real reason is much more mundane. Glycol is cheaper to manufacture and distribute than vegetable oil. If it is better at extracting than vegetable oil, it is going to reduce costs regardless. Speaking personally, I'd rather stick with the vegetable oil. The liquid mixture of annatto seeds and oil/glycol is then treated with a strong alkali. Common examples are sodium hydroxide [32](E 524) or potassium hydroxide (E 525 [33]). Both compounds are used to blacken olives. And both compounds are used extensively in the fruit processing discussed below. Yes, the same substances used in every secondary (high) school chemistry laboratory in the world. The mixture is then evaporated to produce a powder that is about 25% bixin. Other extraction methods employ methanol (an alcohol), acetone (a solvent and precursor compound for BPA manufacture - see chapter five), or hexane.[34] None of these solvents have a designated e number as they are considered processing and/or manufacturing aids. The industry is not obliged to inform as to their use in food processing. Hexane is used across the smorgasbord of 21st century industrial activity. One of its many functions is to extract oils from canola and a soybean seed which means it is of great importance to the GM food industry. As far as the tricksy ice cream is concerned, it contains no real cream at all. So, I think it is safe to assume that the E 160b listed as an ingredient, is also not the real thing. Even if it is, the annatto has likely been subject to the kind of processes outlined above; it will be as far removed from real annatto as Planet Earth is from the heliosphere. The coconut milk is likely to have been heavily processed as per the type of activity hyperlinked here [35]. Any vitamins or other molecules extracted from coconut milk are likely to have their own designated e number. The e number will be the same irrespective of the food the chemicals will have been extracted from. Such are the realities of substantial equivalence. As for the glycerides the manufacturer does not have to state which particular compounds or how much is in the ice cream. These chemicals are outlined in the Food Conspiracy Chorleywood Bread Process book. The parent company for this particular brand of non-ice cream is Unilever. Behind the obvious green and other forms of washing, this is a transnational corporation whose annual turnover is measured in tens of billions of currency units. Sustainability, health and nutrition are not their primary objectives; making cash for themselves, their shareholders and executives is. Finally, on a TV channel (I'm not going to name here) participants blind sample a whole range of processed foods. During the editing for this book the participants were asked to say what they thought of different brands of ice cream. So, naturally enough my interest was piqued. Lo and behold the brand under scrutiny here was selected, which as you can imagine really whetted my appetite.

All of the contestants loved this particular brand, my favourite nugget of verbal enthusiasm being *"wow that is an ice-cream I can sit on the sofa and eat by the bowl load"*. Bearing in mind that these people are supposed to be chefs as well as food and culinary experts, you can forgive me for having a quiet little chuckle as I write this sentence. At the time I was giggling and laughing with somewhat more gusto. For all the wrong reasons you understand it was truly a laugh or cry moment, so I went for the former.

When I put this section together I decided to carry out an impromptu experiment. I took note of the different prices of ice-cream, starting with the cheapest and finishing with the most expensive. I was wondering if I could establish a correlation between price and ice-cream content. The reader should not be surprised to find that I did! There is a steady increase in price all the way to the top of the range. The *"deluxe"* and *"indulgent"* varieties or those which contain *"real chocolate"* or *"real fruit pieces"* mark the steady increase in cost. The peak of the tower is the *"super deluxe ice-cream"* which has the same emulsifiers as listed above but with different stabilisers, flavourings and colourants depending on the type of ice-cream. Which brings us to the crucial point, this most expensive ice-cream has attained the dizzying heights of 23% double cream (according to the label at any rate). All other ice creams have less cream in them and the price drops in direct correlation to the percentage decrease in cream. Aside from varying concentrations of frozen cream all of these ice creams are a mix of water, emulsifiers and the necessary other additives. To my mind, this is not ice cream! I dread to think what kind of quasi- legal shenanigans occurred, how many brown envelopes filled with cash have passed between various grubby hands so that the manufacturers continue to get away with it. And not just with ice cream either! It would be naïve in the extreme to suggest that the industry does not operate in a similar manner with all the food it processes. And just in case you were thinking that somehow this is an isolated example, a rotten egg in the basket if you will, shall we have a look at processed fruit juice? Well yes, why not? After all, it is one of our five a day.

## Selection Three: Fruit Juice

The fruit juices which array the supermarket shelves are invariably tetra packed. The first Tetra Paks appeared in 1954. Their invention and development is credited (if that is the right word) to Erik Wallenberg and Ruben Rausing respectively. To date, The Tetra Pak Company is the largest food packaging organisation in the world. Both the inventors and the company itself are supposed to be what we *"the public"* are meant to look up to as some sort of role model for success. The *"tetra pack"* represents one of many dark and pernicious environmental disasters which blight our planet, a reality which the company has begun to acknowledge. However, the current recycling initiatives do nothing about those Tetra-Paks which reside in landfills or part compose the *"garbage patches"* which are polluting the oceans. Secondly, once you start to dig a little deeper and analyse what terms like *"recycling"* really mean, the picture becomes much less green and sustainable [36]. OK returning to the subject in hand the wonderful world of processed fruit juice. The tetra packs themselves are adorned with statements declaring *"100% pure squeezed"* or *"never from concentrate"* and express with gusto that the juice is *"1 of your 5 a day"*. Genuinely fresh fruit juice is an essential source of vitamins and apart from anything else it tastes great. However, real freshly squeezed juice, that is straight from the fruit, is not what we are discussing here. This section of text grew out of a real conversation which occurred in our household in late 2016. Recently, my girlfriend and I took it upon ourselves to partake of a nightcap (or three) of vodka, cranberry and orange juice topped with lemonade (about 3 parts mixer to 1 part spirit is about right, with crushed ice and a slice of lime). It wasn't a school night so we said with great conviction *"why not?"*

I'm writing about fruit juice because we had a couple of cartons still in the fridge from the festival season of 2016. They were opened at some stage of that summer and we partook of said night cap during November. Now, I had already been writing about additives so I did not expect the juice to be additive free. I fully expect any food that comes in a carton, tin, bottle or packet to have been altered in some way or other. However, when I went to the fridge and picked up both open cartons of fruit juice, I could see that the carton looked as if it had expanded. I assumed that the juice had started fermenting; remember it had been in the fridge for a good 3-4 months and possibly even longer. Here's how two minutes of late night (well early morning) ever so slightly (honest) inebriated conversation went:

**Me:** Hey sweetheart shall we have a vodka drinky drink?

**Girlfriend:** Yes that's an excellent plan.

**Me:** OK let's do that then. I'll check those open cartons of fruit juice, they must have gone by now, it's just as well we have got some more.

At this point, I poured a little orange juice into a glass, smelled it and then tasted and then repeated with the cranberry juice.

**Me:** No way, it's absolutely fine; I wonder if the cranberry is the same, you can check them both as well....

**Girlfriend:** Yep, tastes and smells OK to me...at which point she looked at me and asked: *"How long have they been in the fridge for?"*

**Me:** Between 3 and 6 months

**Girlfriend**: That cannot be right you know. How processed is that then?

**Me:** I have no idea, but I tell you what I'm going to find out and it's going in the book.

Obviously, we had the vodka and mixer combination. The juice was still OK a week later when we finished the last of it off –

without the vodka! I love freshly squeezed juices of all kinds and not always with spirits either. From experience, everyone knows that real fresh and unprocessed orange juice will start to spoil within a couple of days, even kept in the fridge. So, two obvious questions come knocking on the door:

- How do you change real fruit juice into a form which can sit in an open container (albeit sealed and refrigerated) for up to 6 months and show absolutely no sign of spoilage or fermentation?
- How can it be that fresh fruit juice shows no sign of spoilage from the microbes which use the air we breathe as their habitat"?

Clearly, any substance that can resist the highly evolved attentions of airborne microbes must have been altered in some fundamental manner. So what kind of processes [37] is this fruit juice subject [38] to?

Modern fully automated orange juice manufacturing plants can pulp up to 2000 tonnes of oranges every day. The whole orange is put into the machine and as much juice and oil as possible is extracted from the fruit. The skin and most of the pith are separated from the orange fruit itself. The oranges are treated with various acids and agri-chemicals, ensuring every drop of juice is removed from the fruit. Speaking of agri-chemicals the fruit itself is likely to have been sprayed with substances including but limited to organophosphates. [39] Trace quantities of these noted neuro-toxins are likely to be in the juices which sit in our collective fridges. The peel and skin from different fruits is further processed and normally ends up in animal feed. Another conduit for trace concentrations of nasty chemicals to enter the human food chain presents itself. Plenty of evidence exists to buttress the notion that organophosphates can and do induce BSE like symptoms in cattle. On a long enough time line, it is entirely possible that similar symptoms can express themselves in human beings. As far as juice removal is concerned one of the substances employed is gibberellic acid [40] ($C_{19}H_{22}O_6$). As far as I can establish these and the other acids used to process fruit into juice do not have an e number. None of them are listed on the ingredients label either. In the natural world gibberellic is a fungal and plant growth regulator and so is found everywhere in their respective biological kingdoms [41]. Most industrial grade gibberellic acid is obtained from the metabolism of genetically engineered microbes. The microbes are kept in bio-fermenters, i.e. they are stored in a closed system. There is no contact with the outside world on the part of the microbes. The acids also ensure any natural oils are removed from the skin of the fruit. The polysaccharide structural molecules which compose the pith are also broken down. If the juicing mechanism itself is ignored, the juice is by and large fit to be called a freshly squeezed juice because it contains all the substances one would expect a genuinely freshly extracted or squeezed juice to contain. However, things rapidly deteriorate from here. Once collected the freshly squeezed juice is hermetically sealed in a holding tank and the atmosphere is removed. Our atmosphere, the air we breathe, is about 21% oxygen. The gas exists as two oxygen atoms which are chemically bonded to each other. The molecule is highly reactive and combustible. So the oxygen has to be removed before the extracted and treated juice can be stored. Simultaneously, the air that we breathe is replaced with either argon gas or other unreactive gases; a new inert atmosphere is created inside the tank. The *"new atmosphere"* creates an internal environment in which the extracted juice will not spoil. Argon is in group 8 / 18 of the periodic table (the noble gases). This group of molecules is chemically inert meaning they do not react with other substances. It is so stable that it does not react with other elements or compounds. Using argon gas in this way does have proven benefits,[42] but this is not one of them. The replacement argon gas also stops the external air pressure from taking advantage of the pressure drop inside the tank. Have a look at what happens when the air is removed from any solid and hollow object to see what is meant by *"taking advantage"*. As with most industrial processes, the scale is huge. Thousands if not millions of litres of juice can be held inside each tank. The juice itself can be stored for over a year. We have one reason why cartons of fruit juice are available all year round. This may seem to be a fair trade off and at face value, it certainly looks that way. However, as with issue, you can think of, in this world, it just isn't that simple.

De-oxygenating the juice and its immediate environment has one nutritionally catastrophic downside; the process removes the taste of the juice as well as flavor, texture and all the attributes which make a juice, a juice. The fresh juice has been converted into a coloured solution filled with dissolved fructose and pretty much nothing else. It contains no vitamins, minerals, fibre, pectin or any other substances that were present before the juice was processed. Little wonder that campaigns exist to have the statement *"part of your 5 a day removed"* from cartons of processed fruit juice. Within this frame, it is more than reasonable to ask *how can such a drink be termed as fresh in the first place"?* As applied to fruit and vegetables, the Oxford English Dictionary uses *"garden fresh"* or *"newly harvested"* and *"natural"* as well as *"unprocessed"* in its definition of the word *"fresh"*. Even if no other substances were added to the coloured solution, which used to be fruit juice, I fail to see how it can by definition be referred to as fresh. All of the vitamins and minerals are removed, so synthetic copies of the real nutrients are added under the guise of nutrification mentioned above and in chapter one. The originally extracted juice is converted to a sugary solution which is as close to real freshly squeezed juice as The Earth is to Venus. All of the character taste and texture is removed. One of the first tasks is to reinstall some sense of flavor or taste to the solution. This is achieved by means of *"a flavour pack"*. This is a collection of chemicals derived directly from the fruit itself and/or synthetic copies of them. One example is a chemical called ethyl-butyrate [43] ($C_6H_{12}O_2$). [44] This particular substance is an ester. It forms when ethanol (the alcohol) chemically bonds with butyric acid (the organic/carboxylic acid). As a class of compounds, esters are responsible for the flavour, aromatic character and therefore taste of many foods. They also give perfumes and fragrances their characteristic scent. Ethyl-butyrate is responsible for the sweet smell and taste of ripe apples. So, it will be used in apple juice processing. Equivalent esters will be used in the manufacture of other processed fruit juices. The latest regulations stipulate that flavours and aromas removed by the processing can be *"optionally permitted to be restored to fruit juices"*. The producers decide whether to add the ester and whether to declare it on the label of the juice in question. Most of the added esters do not have an e number, they are almost certain to be synthetic forms too. Ethyl-butyrate is very cheap to manufacture, is soluble in many solvents and has uses in cosmetics and plastics. It is also employed as a plasticizer in the cellulose production mentioned in chapter one. These kinds of industrial cross linkage truly are by word of dysfunction and insanity. The fruit processors work with fragrance manufacturers to develop the right flavour for a given juice. It is the ester compounds which add flavour and taste to the juices in question. Ethyl-butyrate is something of a workhorse, but other synthetic esters are used in exactly the same way. For instance, a chemical called methyl butanoate contributes to the flavour of strawberries. A substance called iso-pentyl acetate contributes to the aroma of ripe bananas. These and equivalent synthetic forms are present in these fruit juices. Once again there is no compulsion or requirement for these substances to be declared, so they are not. Do you see made with XYZ artificial ester on your carton of fruit juice? Exactly! Artificial flavour chemicals are added to the concoction to give the illusion of real fruit flavour. Other highly profitable cross linkages exist in fruit and other forms of processing. As was made clear in the introduction, this book will only at best imperceptively scratch the surface of a 3 dimensional object which covers the entire western world. The various food processing conglomerates which compose this object have also put a firm down payment on the remainder of food production on planet Earth too. Collectively, these different vested interests have no need, or more importantly desire, to make any changes that are detrimental to their collective bank balance. The manufacturers are not concerned with making healthy and wholesome fruit juice, they are concerned with maintaining and ideally increasing their profits. Clearly, something has gone wrong with fruit juice. In our nearest supermarket, the price of fresh oranges is prohibitive as compared to a litre of so called fresh orange juice. For us, it is about four times as prohibitive. Our solution is to buy the organic brand when we can and juice up fruits from the *"reduced to clear"* or as we call it *"cheap seats"* section. Failing that we do succumb to financial necessity and purchase the nutrified coloured liquid which should not by any objective benchmark be called fruit juice. The reasons for such a ridiculous state of affairs are myriad and complex, but as always it boils down to one simple reality. It is more profitable as a function of fruit grown and sold for the manufacturers (not the growers or farmers) and supermarket chains to pulp it and turn it into fruit juice in the manner described above than it is to sell more affordable fresh fruit in the first place. The usual retort from the industry is that we *"the population"* are somehow creating the demand and so by association it is our fault that the above techniques are employed.

After processing or import, the cartoned or bottled liquid is sold on as fresh fruit juice. You may be forgiven for thinking that this is the extent of the processing occurring or that no other problems intertwined with it, but I'm afraid to say, again, that you would be wrong.

Once fully de-oxygenated the juice is ready for storage. As a further mechanism to prevent spoilage preservatives are added. They include:

- Sulphur Dioxide (E 220 [45]): An acidic gas which inhibits the activity of enzymes and microbes.

- Sorbic Acid (E 200 [46]) and other sorbates: A series of four preservatives (E 200-203) which prevent the growth of yeast and fungi. They are effective against bacteria but not against other microbes.
- Benzoic Acid (see cellulose in chapter 1) and other benzoates (E 210-219): A family of anti- microbial agents.
- Carbon Dioxide (E 290 [47]): An acidic gas which reduces the pH of the juice itself and inhibits respiration of microbes in an anaerobic atmosphere – i.e. inside the tank.
- Ascorbic acid or Vitamin C (E 300 [48]); Serves as an anti-oxidant and prevents the onset of enzymatic browning [49]. The use and production of Ascorbic acid is outlined in the *"Food Conspiracy book"*.
- Di-methylpyrocarbonate [50]/ di-ethylpyrocarbonate: One of several compounds which curtails the growth of microbes. For example, c.botulinium (see chapter five), which will thrive in an anaerobic environment. It is also used in laboratories to denature specific enzymes.
- Glucono Delta Lactone see chapter 2 (E 575 [51]): A naturally occurring substance which in this application acts as a curing and pickling agent. It also binds up metal ions, stopping them leaching from the tank into the juice.

At this point, a couple of points need to be made which cut right to the chase of this book. Sulphur dioxide is one of the additives which has been used as a preservative for hundreds if not thousands of years. In itself it is not a particularly problematic substance; it is the processing regime itself that is the issue. Citric acid is a natural antioxidant preservative present in citrus fruits and has been used in food preservation and dermatology for many decades. The industry would have you believe that the citric acid is derived from citrus fruits. In the world of 21st century food processing, this is simply not the case. Here, ascorbic acid is derived from sugar beet or sugar cane. The Food Conspiracy book on Chorleywood Bread imparts that these crops provide the sugars which are needed in the processed food industry. Over the next few years, it is highly likely that our species will lurch from one self-inflicted disaster to the next. I drafted that sentence in late 2016 and in mid-September 2017 I see no reason to change my mind. Speaking personally, I would question your grasp and perception of reality if you were to make a different assertion. Within that paradigm and on the current trajectory it is likely that sugar cane and sugar beet crops will categorically fall under the heading genetically modified crops. That is if the industry gets its way. In this direction, any future products which list Vitamin C in its ingredients will contain GMO's or their derivatives. If genetically engineered crops are ever introduced wholesale in the UK we will be looking at a food security disaster that the country may not recover from. The same is true of the wider world too. Secondly, the reader should also note that the phrase "*no artificial colourants or preservatives*" has a bearing on the above list. The above substances can and indeed are framed as "*natural*" but they are produced artificially and are added in precise quantities. Such practices are further exemplified in the "*the Food Conspiracy*" book. They serve the manufacturers by preventing spoilage of the juice and so extend its storage and distribution life. However, they do nothing to improve its nutritional or indeed any other qualities.

From here things become progressively worse. It is now emerging that the pasteurisation and de-aeration of the fruit juice is not absolutely [52] effective. If one takes a second to think about this statement, it is naïve and short sighted to expect otherwise. Micro-organisms (microbes) are loosely defined as any living organism which can only be seen with a microscope of one sort or another. Generally speaking, we are talking about creatures whose entire structure is measured in microns (or micro metres) i.e. $1/1000^{th}$ of a millimetre. As a class of organisms, the microbes have been here on Earth for aeons and have been pivotal in the evolution of life. In about 2 Billion years life on Earth as we know it will be impossible, but likely microbes of one form or another will carry on. In about 4.5 billion years the Earth will be swallowed by the sun when it enters its Red Giant phase. Various microbial species are likely to survive that event too. Microbes are tenacious and adaptable and that means they can set up shop pretty much anywhere. In a very real sense, there are no rules as to where microbes can call their habitat. As the proponents of GMO's are very keen to point out to their opponents, microbes of different species and classes are highly adept at swapping their genetic material. They can and do adapt to pretty much any forces thrown at them and they can do it very quickly. They are known to survive the vacuum of space and travel across the universe in stasis on comets and asteroids. It does not surprise me when I read that various species of fungi and bacteria call the vats in which pasteurised fruit juice is stored home. They have adapted to the anoxic environment and changes in pressure as well as heat which occur during the exchange of oxygen and argon gas. The chemical industry will have developed various agents to kill them off, which the manufacturers will purchase, employ and then tell us that everything is OK. Consequently, we will be ingesting even more unnecessary chemicals as a result of food processing. Equally, the microbes will evolve to deal with agents designed to kill them (they always do) and the whole cycle will continue. And further processing will remove any by-products of such biochemical activity. Again notions of nutrition and sustainable food production are sacrificed on the altar of profit and industrial cross linkage.

## Selection Four: Sauces and Dips

The essential point with condiments is that most of them can be made at home. Some are harder to make than others. For instance, making tomato ketchup uses large amounts of tomatoes and it takes hours to make even a modest amount of sauce. Obviously, cost and time begin to factor into proceedings so we still buy tomato sauce. We do make our own:

- Hummus
- Guacamole
- Tartare Sauce. (OK - we use bought mayonnaise as the base)
- Curry Pastes
- Stir Fry and Asian Cooking Sauces
- Garlic Mayonnaise. (As above but the garlic is fresh)
- Andalouse Sauce
- Pesto
- Relishes. (OK - the ketchup and purees are bought)
- Mushroom and other pates

Truly, hummus is really easy to make. All you need is chick peas, garlic, tahini, lemon juice, a few generous measures of olive oil, paprika and cumin. You can add chopped sweet peppers and any vegetable or spice that you like. All you need to do is soak and cook the chick peas as required, chop up the garlic, grind the spices in a pestle and mortar (how pleased are we to have one of those?) and put everything in a mixing bowl. We have a potato masher and hand held electric blitzing devices. Mash up the mixture and then gently use the electric blitzer until all the ingredients are combined into a thick sauce. Adjust quantities and flavour to your preferences, let the hummus sit for a while and that is it. The making takes about 30 minutes. You just need to allow time for soaking and cooking of the chick peas. Why is it worth it?

This is the ingredients list of a typical brand of shop bought hummus:

- Cooked chick peas (54%)
- Water
- Sesame Seed paste (12%)
- Rapeseed/canola oil (I love to see it called canola oil instead)
- Concentrated Lemon juice (3%)

- Garlic puree
- Salt
- Preservative: Potassium Sorbate

Well, there is not too much *"bad stuff"* in there, but I'm willing to bet that the chick pea content of the hummus I make is somewhere between 90 and 95%, plus there is no added water. Canola oil is mentioned in the *"Food Conspiracy"* book. The oil is likely to be derived from plants grown from genetically engineered seeds and under current EU law there is no obligation to declare either way. Quelle surprise? The manufacturers don't. We do not use the minimum of tahini paste, garlic puree or concentrated lemon juice. We use the juice from a lemon, chopped garlic and the tahini comes in a glass jar which is only *"roasted and pulped sesame seeds"*. Our hummus is almost all chick peas and tahini made with the best fresh and unprocessed ingredients we can afford. The same is true of all the examples below. Leaving all other issues aside the hummus we make just tastes nicer and it freezes well too. Clearly a no brainer!

As for guacamole, the biggest problem you have is finding ripe avocados. Generally, you need to buy them and leave them to ripen for a few days. Then all you do is scoop out the fruit. Afterwards plant the seed where nature might take its course, ditto with ANY fresh vegetable that you buy. We add some chopped tomatoes, chopped red onion, garlic, fresh lemon juice, (from a lemon) and stir it all in together. You ought to make only what you need each time, cover it up and refrigerate. If you make too much it will oxidise and turn black. If you are going to make a bulk amount make sure you freeze it properly. Why is it worth it? This is the ingredients list of a typical brand of Shop bought guacamole:

- Avocado (70%)
- Single cream
- Tomato

- Onion
- Sugar
- Concentrated lime juice
- Coriander
- Anti-oxidant – Ascorbic acid
- Chilli
- Garlic Puree
- Salt
- Rapeseed oil (Canola PLEASE!)
- Rice starch
- Dried red chilli
- Chilli powder

This guacamole is 70% avocado and that is likely to be the case. Even so, it may not be fresh, especially when one considers the lovely concoctions that *"nature seal"* (see chapter two) and their ilk are doing to ostensibly fresh fruits and vegetables. The Introducing GMO's book discusses how tomatoes are treated by the food industry, it is likely that avocados are treated and subjected to similar chemical processes. The other ingredients are likely to be real as well, but, as chapter two imparts, real does not mean fresh. The tomato and onion are likely to have been treated with a preservative and could easily be several weeks old. The guacamole we make is a deep green colour and has a real tang and bite; this shop bought form was a pale insipid green colour, with the taste to boot. We also do not add oil, anti-oxidants or any dried ingredients or starch from grains. If I want extra starch I'll make a risotto!

Tartare sauce is even easier to make than guacamole. All you need is the best quality mayonnaise you can afford, ideally you can make your own but that is not really an option for us. The section on eggs in chapter one explains why we avoid the *"reduced fat"* or *"light varieties"*. These are generally even more processed than the regular brands and contain less egg. So, if you cannot make your own, get hold of the best regular brands your budget allows. Scoop out a couple of large dollops of mayonnaise into a bowl and add enough gherkins and capers to completely fill the mayonnaise. We use between 100-200g capers and about the same mass of gherkins. Both are finely chopped and stirred into the mayonnaise with a large sprinkling of Tarragon. Why is it worth it? This is the ingredients list of a typical brand of Shop bought tartare sauce:

- Rapeseed oil (its canola oil) 60%
- Water.
- Spirit vinegar.
- Glucose – fructose syrup.
- Free range egg yolk (5.3%)
- Capers (2.3%)
- Gherkins (2.1%)
- Salt.
- White wine vinegar
- Modified maize (corn) starch
- Shallots (0.5%)
- Onions
- Acidity regulator- lactic acid and citric acid
- Dijon Mustard (0.2%) – water, brown mustard seeds, spirit vinegar, salt (preservative potassium meta-bi-sulphite) Acid (citric acid)
- Flavourings – contain mustard
- Parsley
- Thickeners – guar gum and xanthan gum

The tartare sauce we make is made from the regular mayonnaise mentioned in chapter one. So, aside from those ingredients, our tartare contains only chopped capers and gherkins, some tarragon and maybe some lemon or lime zest. That is it.

I could go on ad infinitum (forever), but I think the point has been well and truly made. Similar reasoning lays behind our household making the pastes and sauces mentioned above. All you need to do is get a recipe and fresh ingredients and you can do your bit to avoid processed sauces. It really is not difficult or challenging, truly it isn't. You will get some control back over what you are feeding yourself and family. The base for many Asian dishes is ginger, chilli and garlic cooked down in water. You can then add spinach, and kale, coconut paste or milk, other herbs, depending on what you are making. Why is the extra chopping and cooking worth it? Well, this is the ingredients list for a typical brand of shop bought, (produced in the Far East) hoy sin sauce:

- Water.
- Sugar.
- Vegetables (8%) – mixed peppers, onions, carrots.
- Modified Maize (corn) Starch (see chapter three).
- Tomato Puree.
- Pineapple Pieces (1.5%).
- Rice Vinegar.
- Salt.
- Acidity Regulators – acetic acid (vinegar), citric acid, (discussed in *"the Food Conspiracy"* book)
- Soya sauce extract, (water, soya beans, wheat, salt).
- Salted Plums, (plums salt).
- Ginger.
- Garlic.
- Colour – plain caramel.
- Soya oil.
- Herb.
- Stabiliser – xanthan gum [53]/ E 415 [54] (Discussed in the book *"Food Conspiracy - What Happened To Our Bread? The Chorleywood Bread Process"*).
- Spice.

The glaringly obvious point to make is that the overwhelming majority of this particular sauce is sugar and water, the next 8%

is the vegetables and another 1.5% is the pineapple. Other curry pastes, pickles, chutneys and sauces have slightly different combinations of the same ingredients. All have water as the top ingredient, so most of what you are buying is water. You can keep buying packet sauces, or you can cook down some chopped garlic, ginger and chilli add some fresh or ground spices and other ingredients as appropriate. We have also stopped buying cheaper brands of soy sauce. We have managed to offset the extra cost against the savings made by using fresh (ish) ingredients to make the paste and sauce base. The soy sauce we used to buy contains the following ingredients:

- Water
- Sugar
- Soy sauce extracts (9% - water soya bean, wheat and salt)
- Salt
- Colour – Plain Caramel
- Acidity regulator – lactic acid
- Preservative – potassium sorbate

This liquid ought not to be described as a soy sauce. Why? Well, just as with the ice cream outlined above, it contains no real soybean sauce, it is an extract and some caramel to give it the right colour. The rest of this sauce is water and sugar, not exactly the real deal. The brand we buy now is *"naturally brewed"* costs about four times as much as the previous example and has only four ingredients:

- Water
- Soybeans
- Wheat
- Salt

It is made from fermented soy beans and because it contains no added preservatives it will spoil relatively quickly, which is why it is going on tonight's Thai green curry! There is one giant fly in the dark tangy liquid. Soybeans were the first commercially grown Genetically Modified food crop. It never occurred to the agencies behind GM crops to keep their creations separate from the crops which already existed. Under the banner of substantial equivalence (see chapter two) they never even considered it. The biotech and chemical industries which drive GMO's never conceived the level of resistance to their wholly unnecessary crops. Sadly, in 2017, it is almost impossible to absolutely guarantee that any soybeans or their products are GM free, even if the label says so. The European wing of Kikkoman soy sauce is at great pains to state *"Kikkoman takes great care to ensure that only high quality ingredients are used in its natural production process. That's why all Kikkoman products manufactured in The Netherlands are produced exclusively with non-GMO soybeans"*. The glass jar I am looking at now says *"manufactured in the Netherlands"* so I should be resting easy. Except I'm not, and why is that? Well, because products can be labelled GM free even if they contain GM ingredients. There is no compulsion on the manufacturers to state that their product contains GM ingredients. This sauce is likely to contain some ferment derived from GM crops. The company in Europe is very keen to demonstrate its GM free credentials [55]. I also have to say that for taste and flavour (the clue I guess is in the brand name) this more expensive brand knocks the socks off the previous sauce, now why is that I wonder? Could it be that the sauce is made from fermented soy beans and nothing else? As for the sauces made outside of the EU, the picture is much less rosy. The manufacturers do use a mix of GM and non-GM soya beans, with the relative portion of each being subject to their discretion

## Selection Five: Cider

It may seem counter intuitive to end this chapter by writing about an alcoholic drink, but it does tick all the boxes. The label of our most commonly purchased cider clearly says the cider is made from *"a blend of apples"*, which is reflected in the price. I have developed a penchant for home-made wine, in part because

I have the good fortune to be able to pick the fruit from the trees and hedgerows where I live. With this fruit, I make various forms of red wine. The only real concessions to *"processing"* are the concentrated (the concentrate itself) grape juice and the potassium sorbate preservative. The refined sugar has been replaced with an un-refined organic brand. The fruit comes from the brambles and trees and is fermented with yeast and then settled and cleared with finings. The whole process converts fruit into wine using these ingredients and yeast, with the appropriate amount of water – and that is it. The core reason we started buying *"real cider"* is because in cheap brands it is not predominantly apples which are fermented into cider. Almost all budget brands of cider are made from fermented apple concentrate, corn starch syrup, high fructose corn syrup (see chapter seven) and a plethora of apple flavourings and/or enhancers thereof. The resulting brew is then diluted with water until the required alcohol concentration is reached. A dash of malic acid [56] (E 296 [57]) is often added to give the concoction an extra kick or bite. It is more acidic than citric acid. It is used as a preservative and it slows the growth of yeast by reducing the pH of fermenting liquids. It is likely but not certain the malic acid used in food production comes from a GM source. The list of ingredients on the cider we used to buy is:

- Fermented apple juice
- Fermented glucose syrup
- Water
- Sugar
- Carbon dioxide
- Acid E 270 [58](lactic acid [59]) E 330 (citric acid)
- Anti-oxidant E 224 [60] (sulphites) – potassium meta-bi-sulphite [6]

Much of the glucose and glucose syrup used in the food industry is derived from corn, which is almost certain to be a GM variety. It is not even glucose from apples. At present opposition to GM crops is well entrenched across the EU, obviously, I hope that such resistance intensifies. Yet, imports of GM crops for animal feed are allowed here in Europe. Plus, GM corn is grown in Spain, the only EU country which commercially grows GM crops for the human food chain. Irrespective of the issues concerning GM crops overall and GM corn in particular; the point is that a healthy amount of the alcohol in cheap cider does not come from fruit, let alone apples. On that basis alone it cannot by definition be called cider and this particular brand came in a plastic bottle. So, given the absolute criminality ensuing with plastics in the oceans we have switched to a brand which comes in a glass bottle. The glass is properly recycled. As for the cider we now drink, it is still a blend of different apple juices, but it contains no syrup or added sugar (as far as we know). Aside from these differences it the same as the previous brand.

As I wrote at the beginning of this chapter, these are stupid almost pointless choices to make. They truly do represent a sticking plaster on a growing, festering and gangrenous wound. People make such choices because they are the right ones to make. For those of us who call themselves activists, progressives or campaigners, or dare I say it even socialists, those who or are concerned (if not flat out terrified) about the state of things, we make such choices in the hope that other people will begin to follow the example. The people of the Pacific islands are doing everything they can to deal with rising sea levels. They have not caused climate change but they are suffering the consequences. In all likelihood in the very near future, their islands will be submerged under salt water. Yet to the best of their ability the population continue to install solar panels and wind turbines. If they are leading by that kind of example, but are still going to lose their homes, we in the west can make the right individual choices as best we can. This is occurring as the US government and its allies try to stoke up even more global tension, this time against China and North Korea. Doing your bit, so to speak has its place and it must be applauded. I am under no illusions; if we really want to avoid processed food then the concluding point made in chapter three is the only real long term answer.

# Chapter Five: How Did It Come To This?

The industrial and agricultural revolutions changed every aspect of life in 19th century Britain. Almost immediately the wider world followed suit. Before these game changing events, it would be fair to say that the meagre revenue generated from farming stayed within the community which produced it. This was no romantic agrarian utopia, a lot of the majority of the population was (even by today's deteriorating standards), deplorable to say the least. Nevertheless, growers had a real connection to the land they worked and the animals they reared, as did members of the wider community. Putting it mildly Life was undoubtedly hard and brutal; short and precarious. It was garnished with extra dashes of abuse and was riddled with injustice. Most of us today would find such circumstances intolerable. Others, including myself, impart with good reason that nothing much has changed. For the growers of 19th century Britain the yields from the fields would have been significantly less than today. If yields were the only way to measure agricultural productivity and long term sustainability we would be in a much better food security position than we are. Clearly, other factors come into measurements of agricultural yield. For instance, the productivity of mono-cultured agriculture is only maintained by the employment of oil based chemical fertilisers. A consummate depletion of aquifers and a criminal waste of water to irrigate these cash crops has been occurring since the 1950's. Despite its noble intentions, the green revolution has now set a precedent whereby *"big agriculture"* and other oligarchs are now mining water that has been left undisturbed for hundreds of thousands if not millions of years. Our world is running out of fresh water and our species is facing an agricultural time bomb, of its own systemic making. I am writing of a geopolitical explosive device born of vanity, ego, greed, theft, exploitation, abuse, waste and environmental destruction. This device is very likely to supplant the horrors of part forgotten events like the Irish potato famine, the Russian Famine of 1921-22 and the Ukrainian famine of 1932-33 into the current global context. The Irish potato famine is to date the worst humanitarian disaster to ever befall peacetime Europe. The cause of the famine is rooted in biology and a lack of variation in the potato crop itself. A largely avoidable catastrophe was exacerbated by British government policy toward the Irish people. Transferring the twisted mentality of the Reverend Thomas Malthus into an instrument of British foreign policy the Irish rural poor, in particular, were deliberately starved. And starve they most certainly did. About a million people were killed unnecessarily and up to three million more were forced to migrate to the emerging urban slums of Britain and the United States. Malthus should be stripped of his religious credentials and history ought to view him as the racist sociopath, misanthropist and psychopath he so clearly was. Against this backdrop, the European powers and the rising US colossus, were between them making brutal war in foreign lands and against each other. Again I can argue that not very much has changed since the mid-1840's. Clearly, such system inflicted and so avoidable atrocity, destruction, murder and genocide is carrying on unabated in 2017. For instance, take a look at the deliberate policies concerning Yemen, the climate basis for events in Syria and Darfur and the additional unfolding crime against humanity in the Horn of Africa and it is difficult to come to any other conclusion. These are not isolated examples. Such crimes have been occurring for all my life, further back into history and absolutely nothing is being done to stop them happening in the first place. Truly, the lessons of history have been deliberately ignored. In a world which has between only 60 [1] and 100 [2] harvests left it is a safe bet that the current agricultural system and those it supports is very much living on borrowed time. The food produced in pre-industrial Britain would fall under *"artisan"* or *"traditional"*. Nutritionally speaking the food was light years away from the processed fare on offer today. There just wasn't much variety, or very much to go around, the diet was monotonous and crop failure was a constant fear.

Human beings are the only animals on the planet that routinely process the food they eat. At some point between 3,500 and 2,500 years ago in various locations *"money and coin"* began to integrate itself into our relationships with each other. Direct food adulteration has been occurring for over 3000 years and can with some justification be linked to the first use of money as a form of universal exchange. Both the evolution of money and the Neolithic revolution which preceded it occurred in different regions and for different reasons around the world. Established preservation techniques have been with us since human beings first found themselves with surpluses of food. The techniques include salting, smoking and fermentation. These *"traditional"* or *"artisan"* (read beneficial) food processing techniques exist for two basic purposes. The first is to make food easier for us to digest. The second is to preserve and store it, normally for the *"lean times"*. Irrespective of how they are organised, there are plenty of highly nutritious and well preserved processed foods in the different food groups. Equally important the food produced by traditional or artisan means results in revenue which is ploughed back into the farm, community or cooperative it came from. Such activity is alive and thriving but not to anything like the degree that it could be and should be. Traditional activity has been largely superseded by the prolific use of various synthetic additives and processing aids. Food produced by modern intensive methods is certainly not as nutritious as it should be and as for being more easily digested, I guess it depends on who you ask. In the 21st century, we live in a world whose very fabric of organisation is well on the way to complete disintegration. One component of the total collapse most of humanity faces is the justifiably eviscerated *"western diet"* [3] and everything it represents. The modern world does not have the monopoly on adding chemicals to food. For the past several hundred years substances which may be toxic have been routinely added to the food human beings eat. Whether it is for reasons of profit, or out of a genuine necessity human beings have been altering (i.e. processing) food since we learned how to utilise fire. Before the 20th century, chemicals were routinely added to food deemed fit for human consumption, for example:

- Strychnine [4] ($C_{21}H_{22}N_2O_2$ - rodent poison) and sulphuric acid ($H_2SO_4$ [5]) were added to ales to give them an extra kick and to mask signs of spoilage. It also meant that more beer could be produced from a given quantity of hops.
- Water was routinely added to milk which increased its volume. Yellow, powdered [6] lead chromate, ($PbCrO_4$ [7]), was mixed in to provide the illusion of richness and to imitate the presence of cream
- The quintessentially British mug of tea was once laced with red coloured *"rock gypsum"* (hydrated calcium sulphate - $H_4CaO_6S$ [8]). It was supposed to improve the colour, taste and texture of the brew. Today Gypsum is used in extensively in construction as well as in the manufacture of cement, plaster of Paris, paper and synthetic rubber.
- The nascent confectionery industry used a substance called *"red lead"* to colour its boiled sweets. Red lead is lead (IV) oxide [9] ($PbO_2$) and is insoluble in water. The compound will partially dissolve in nitric and sulphuric acid. It also reacts with hydrochloric acid and liberates chlorine gas as it does so. Concentrated hydrochloric acid is found in the human stomach. I think the reader can guess what happened next. The pungent farts might be amusing, but the reaction of the gas with the moisture in the colon forms a weak solution of hydrochloric acid, which would have caused irritation of varying degrees of severity. Ouch! Red lead was also used in the manufacture of safety matches. In the 1970's the oxide was the adsorbing surface for sulphur dioxide ($SO_2$). This acidic gas is one of the main culprits of acid rain.
- The spices most of us take for granted were shockingly expensive as compared to those available today. They were

combined with dust, ground nut shells, sand, stones and seeds, or combinations thereof depending on the spice in question.

- Copper sulphate ($CuSO_4$) or blue vitriol, is including its other toxic effects, a very powerful emetic (induces vomiting). That did not stop it being added to canned vegetables to provide an illusion of freshness and colour.

- Salicylic (hydro-benzoic) acid ($C_7H_6O_3$) is a natural carboxylic (carbon based) acid, which is present naturally many plants and their fruits and vegetables. It was used as a preservative but excessive consumption can lead to symptoms including asthma, hives, [10] headaches, stomach pain and swelling of varying severity. Today intolerance and allergic reactions mean that its use as a preservative is generally discouraged. This only occurred because of the kind of laws mentioned below and not because of concern over negative health impacts. As a class of compounds, the salicylates are used extensively in cosmetics, for treating acne and in making dyes for the textile and clothing industries. The salicylates are of great importance to the pharmaceutical industry. They are used as precursor compounds for many different medicines. Arguably the most well-known salicylic based compound is aspirin.

- Borax (di-sodium tetra-borate) is a hugely important substance for the manufacture of glass and ceramics. In food its main utilities were as a preservative, to provide extra texture (whatever that means) and to give flexibility to cooked foods. It also facilitates the dissolving of metal oxides and so is equally important for any process that requires metals as end products. It produces chemicals which are used as fungicides in paint, fire retardant plastics and in petrochemicals. It is still used in detergents and as an antiseptic in medicine. It is a recognised carcinogen whose use as a food preservative is banned in the US, EU and the western world. Boric acid is present naturally in fruits, nuts, leafy vegetables, wine, cider and beer.

- Formaldehyde ($H_2CO$) also known as methanal is another natural substance found everywhere in the plant and animal kingdom. It is a highly pungent gas which readily dissolves in water. It is also an acidic gas when it dissolves the pH of a given solution will decrease. Formaldehyde is so that it does not exist in a pure form. In industry, a substance called Formalin acts as the main formaldehyde source. Formaldehyde is liberated from the solution and is used to manufacture plastics, fertilisers, textiles, fungicides, cosmetics and household cleaning products. It was used extensively, as a food preservative and pickling agent, with potentially fatal results. It can cause symptoms ranging from mild vomiting to stomach cramps, renal (kidney failure) and coma. In 2004 it was designated as *"carcinogenic to humans"* by the World Health Organisation (WHO).

These are not isolated examples. Over the last couple of centuries or so, hundreds if not thousands of individual examples of this kind of adulteration present themselves. If one is feeling generous and accommodating (which I don't), you can argue that we simply did not know that lead is a highly potent neurotoxin (amongst its other terrible biological impacts). This does not excuse or divert from the simple reality that the adulterations were made to increase profits. Today the industry is using a whole range of synthetic and artificial compounds to achieve exactly the same aim. In the 21st century, thousands of individual compounds exist in processed foods. It is naïve in the extreme to suppose no possibility of long term negative biological impact, for the hundreds of millions of people, including you and I, who ingest them on an almost daily basis. Remember that this writing focuses on the western world. It is highly likely that plenty of substances banned or regulated here in the west are not likely to be so in the rest of the world.

## Origins of modern UK Food Law

Before 1875 no enforced law existed to prevent the unfettered adulteration of the food eaten by most of the population. In 1820 the sale of some known poisons was regulated or made illegal. However, most of them were available if you knew where to look. In addition, plenty of pharmacists were distributing known poisons on demand. This began to change as the following time line of events unfolded. For instance, the sale of arsenic became controlled under the auspices of the 1851 Pharmacy act. In 1868 a follow up pharmacy act included the regulation of strychnine, potassium cyanide and ergot. Equivalent legislation came into being later on in the US. By the time of the machine gun massacre of North American Indian women, children and the final extermination of the last great Indian nation, at Wounded Knee in 1890, about 30 states in the US had adopted some form of pharmacy law. Before such acts, there was no analytical method to determine the presence of such substances in the food most people were eating. The law in the UK before 1851 was in effect toothless and redundant. As far as food was concerned nothing short of a poisoner free for all existed. This unforgiving reality began to change in the early 19th century. Arguably most of the credit for modern food legislation can be granted to a German chemist called Frederick Accum. He arrived in London in the late 18th century and by 1820 was acutely aware of how severe food adulteration was in London. It soon became obvious that the same issues were occurring in every industrial centre in Britain. In 1820 Accum published [11] a book called *"A treatise on adulterations of food and culinary poisons"*. The book sold out in a few months and was subsequently published in the US before the end of the year. The work was translated into German in 1822 and consequently, it became a best seller in his home country and the rest of Europe too. The book argues that adulteration was endemic across industrial revolution Britain. It also became clear that such criminal activity was not limited to food poisoning either. However, it was the altering of food with chemicals that really ground Accum's gears. And based on the slivers of information I have found out, I can't say I blame him. He argued that food adulteration was so severe that in the name of public health, it ought to be seen as a criminal offence. I have no problem with such notions. The last sections in this book demonstrate that similar charges ought to be levied against those behind the comparable practices employed today. Frederick Accum clearly had a sense of injustice and questioned the "*way of things*". He said of British law "*The man who robs a fellow subject of a few shillings on the highway is sentenced to death'. Yet, 'he who distributes a slow poison to the whole community escapes unpunished'.* Again more foundation for stating that nothing much has changed in the modern world.

One practice which really caught Accum's beady eye was tea and coffee. Except, that what was being sold to the "*working classes*" could not be described as either tea or coffee. By 21st century standards, the drinking of tea and coffee was a hugely expensive undertaking; it was something of a status symbol. Real tea was unaffordable for most people in 19th century Britain. Any leftover tea leaves and coffee grains were sold on by the coffee and tea houses of Britain; it was then treated by chemical means. The objective being to make the brew produced from the spent leaves and beans look as close to the real thing as possible. The leftovers were boiled in a solution of iron sulphate ($FeSO_4$) and sheep faeces, hmmmm, lovely! During boiling the brew was coloured with one or more of the following:

- Iron Cyanide (Prussian blue)
- Copper acetate (Verdigris)
- Logwood [12] dye
- Tannins
- Carbon black AKA soot

This was then sold on as tea or coffee. I assume that the people who drank this appalling and noxious mix had no real concept of what the real thing tasted like. Assuming they got past what must have been a revolting stench I hope they took one sip and left well alone. Other strategies included adding dried plant leaves which were anything but tea. As for other forms of coffee, it could be mixed with other beans, chicory, sand and gravel. Chicory itself was often mixed up with roasted root vegetables and caramelised sugar, to give the characteristic colour of black coffee. The brews were not necessarily poisonous but by any standards, such practices surely constitute fraud and therefore theft. In modern parlance, we might refer to them as alt-tea and alt-coffee. As Accum carried on his analytical foray into early 18th century food adulteration he certainly found some pretty nasty chemicals. He found various salts of lead, copper and iron present across most of the foods and drinks that most people in urban Britain ingested. He found mercury salts in boiled sweets plus he found salts of tin in vinegar and so it went on. Crucially Accum had the courage to name and shame those who were selling such altered foods. Which as you can imagine made him really popular! He was attacked and discredited by his peers in much the same way as those of us who speak out today are vilified. That is by any means necessary, no trick was too low, nefarious or below the belt. Accum was hounded and brayed everywhere he went and in 1821 he had no choice but to leave Britain. Nothing was done concerning the state of food adulteration or its consequences, for another 3 decades. I wonder how many lives were blighted and cut short by an elite and business class that exists only to enrich itself? Sound familiar? It does to me.

In the 1830's a politician called Thomas Wakley [13] who was also editor for *"The Lancet"* medical journal began picking up where Accum had left off. He was well embedded with the Chartist [14] movement of the mid-19th century and fought that particular cause long and hard during his political and parliamentary career. Think of what a real left wing political organisation might stand for and you'll have an idea of what the Chartists [15] were all about. They carried on the militancy of the Luddite movement which preceded them. During the course of researching this book I came across this potentially prophetic relevant quote, *"when robots take our jobs, just remember the Luddites"*. I am no expert on ICT, robotics, artificial intelligence or technology by any means. However, the level of potential job losses that automation looks set to cause is but one example of the global socio-economic upheaval which, on the current path, is just around the corner. From what I can work out an equivalent set of circumstances which faced The Luddites in the early 19th century, looks set to present themselves in the very near future. Those who were at the sharp end of such upheaval were more prepared to fight for their rights than those who are set to suffer the most in the very near future. The Luddite rebellion of 1811-13 was violently put down by the British ruling class. Their legacy continues to this day and the Chartist movement is perhaps the next step in the story of organised global resistance to the objectives of the agency we would today term the elite. Across the pond, a militant movement called the Molly Maguires [16] had equivalent aims for the US working classes. The Maguires were also particularly active in Ireland. The Chartists sought freedom for the majority from the shackles of state repression and the exploitation of so many people in 19th century Britain. They sought to achieve this through petitioning, mass movements, strikes, occupations and demonstrations. Societal change was to be achieved by any and all non-violent means available to them. Many supporters and activists were jailed for their trouble. Again it is difficult to see that things have meaningfully improved since their time. Thomas Wakley was to all and intents and purposes the complete opposite of the thoroughly repugnant Thomas Malthus. Wakley worked in conjunction with Arthur Hill Hassall,[17] who was a London based doctor. His field was immunology and molecular biology and he was one of the true pioneers in both disciplines. Between them, they carried on where Frederick Accum had been compelled by opposition to leave Britain. A key indicator of Hassall's drive and passion can be exemplified by his 1855 book *"Food and its Adulterations"*. The text represents the result of years of hard campaigning, against an emerging industry which was knowingly poisoning whole populations in the name of profit. A key development in the analysis of adulterated food was the light microscope. Hassall, who gained his doctorate from Oxford University, was well versed in the techniques of microscopy. It was the microscope which enabled Hassall to begin to properly study food samples. It became very easy to establish what was present in a given sample. It became obvious as to what was an adulterant and that which was not. The relative proportions of *"adulterant"* and *"non-adulterant"* could be established. For instance, analysis by microscope established the presence of mites and other insects in flour, sugar and similar dry and/or powdered foods available at the time. These works gained the attention of Wakley who was seeking to legislate against the kind of practices which fell under the banner *"food adulteration"*. As far as Wakley and Hassell were concerned it must have been clear to those in the know what was going on; the question was how to prove it. In the early 1850's about 3000 individual food samples were analysed and the names and addresses of all vendors were dutifully and methodically recorded. The results and names of sellers were published with Wakley taking the financial hit for the inevitable legal costs. The team work carried out by Wakley and Hassell re-established everything that Accum had found out and then some, with extra bells too. In 1855 Hassall published his findings under his own name and detailed the names and addresses of each offender next to what was found in the *"food"* they sold. Then as now, it was established that adulteration was the norm and not the exception. And the scene was set for the incarnation of modern British food law.

- In 1860 the very first Food Adulteration act was passed.
- In 1872 an amended version was passed taking on board the shortfalls of the 1860 version.
- In 1874 the Society of Public Analysts (SPA) was founded.

A nationwide organisation set up for the sole purpose of analysing food samples irrespective of their source.

- In 1875 the sale of food and drugs act was passed this occurred largely as a result of findings by the SPA.
- In 1879 the Sale of food and drugs act was further amended.
- In 1879 the Margarine act came into force.
- In 1887 the original 1860 act was further amended.

By the late 19th century, the willful chemical adulteration of food in Britain became illegal and offenders were liable to prosecution by fine and/or prison. This was not a concession given by a benign establishment that had seen the error of its ways or made a mistake. All offenders from the manufacturers all the way down the line to the final seller knew exactly what was going on. They fought viciously against every move made against them. If they were so concerned about *"public health"*, at the very least they would have taken on board the findings of Frederick Accum, but they didn't, they did the exact opposite. Consequently, several decades more suffering was inflicted on the people of Britain. Hmmmm, well, once again, it still sounds all too familiar to me! The above types of legislation pertaining to food safety are exactly the kind of statutes that are likely to be in the Brexit firing line, when or if, the UK formally leaves the EU.

## Origins of Food Law in the US

The first US food law to be passed with anything approaching teeth was the 1906 Food and Drug Act. Later, in the same year, the meat inspection act came into force. Before them, in Europe, the US and the wider western world, no regulation existed concerning what could be added to the food people were eating. Just as in Britain, across the Atlantic absolutely no consideration or regard was given to direct impacts on human health. No regard was given to the sources or production techniques of the compounds in question, the producers and vendors fought tooth and nail to keep it that way too. No talk of *"environmental impact"* or *"public health"* was heard, these phrases simply did not exist. Well, they don't in the corridors of power; they do in the land of humanity and empathy, love and logic where I live. When it comes to the bank balance all other concerns become secondary. Wowee zowee, there is that familiar position all over again, go figure! In the late 19$^{th}$ and early 20$^{th}$ century, hundreds of compounds which are now banned (in the western world) were used liberally to keep processed foods visually appealing and to cover the signs of rotting. The food legislation of 1906 came into force with a federal mandate to enforce it. Successive US governments have sought to undermine such laws with perhaps the current unstable administration being the most demented. Even by western standards, the Trump presidency looks set to become by far the worst offender. A huge credit for the 1906 statutes has to be given to Dr Harvey Washington Wiley, who was the chief chemist for the US Department of Agriculture (DOA). If you will, he was a US version of Accum, Wakley and Hassall. For instance, he is known to have stated publicly that the American people were being *"steadily"* and *"deliberately"* poisoned by the chemicals that were being added to food in the US. This assertion was made possible by the actions of a group of fit and healthy young men. Sadly Wiley was something of a sexist and he did not believe women to be as capable as men. In any studies or research, he had direct control of women did not even get a look in. In the largely male dominated world of early 20$^{th}$ century science, Wiley was not alone in such borderline, if not flat out misogyny. Nevertheless, the experiment became a pivotal landmark in the implementation of US food law.

In 1902 Wiley asked for 12 male volunteers from the DOA. The experimental regime was devastating in its simplicity and flat out danger to the health of the individuals concerned. Wiley seriously believed that physically and mentally women would just not be up to what he had in mind. The experimental brief was simple; the volunteers would eat only what they were prescribed by Dr Wiley. The idea was to demonstrate what happens to erstwhile healthy people when they ate the food available at the time. The experiment was also carried out in the public domain because Wiley wanted the public to see the results for themselves. He wanted the population to push for changes in the law themselves, another proposition that I have no problem with. In fact, it is something I actively encourage. The experiment ran for 12 months. Yum yum, chowing down on a diet composed mainly of processed food, where do I sign up for that then? More recently others have chosen to do exactly the same thing (albeit for less time) and for opposite reasons. I would say to such people, on you go, sign up for the Darwin awards if you must, but you are missing the point. Most of the additives should not be there. I would also ask why you are wasting your time and potentially damaging the health of those around you, trying to justify the activities of an industry that only exists to the benefit of itself. Certainly, I'm with Wiley, Accum, Wakley and Hasall, on this issue, all the way. In 1902 the 12 volunteers were fed food containing measured doses and quantities of the substances in the food people were eating at the time. For good reason, the volunteers became known as the *"poison squad"*. The volunteers pledged for one year to eat only the diet prescribed by Dr Wiley. There were two disclaimers. First, a person could stop eating if they became sick or unwell as a result of the diet. Second, in the event of death, the right to sue was waived. The members of the poison squad were fed food containing amongst other substances:

- Borax
- Sulphuric Acid
- Saltpetre (see below)
- Formaldehyde
- Copper sulphate
- Benzoic and dozens of other organic acids.
- Diamorphine (Heroin)

- Prussic Acid (hydrogen cyanide)

The squad was eating the complete range of food adulterants used at the time and in the same concentrations as being eaten by the majority of the US population. The food lobbyists of the time fought tooth and nail to suppress what was predictably happening to the health of the individuals concerned. As with his European counterparts Wiley was vilified and on more than several occasions, he was ordered by his own agency (the DOA) not to publicise his findings. My goodness, there it is again, that familiar position! My word one could be forgiven for thinking there is a historical pattern identical to the behaviour going on today, in the 21$^{st}$ century. Get away........you're making it up!

In 1906 the US Food, Drug and insecticide administration came into being, whose name was then shortened to the Food and drug Administration (FDA). The FDA is the regulatory body which, theoretically, determines which substances and in what quantities are allowed in the food the US population eats. In the late 19$^{th}$ century and early 20$^{th}$ century, Wiley continually exposed the degree to which this community was being poisoned by the chemicals added to processed food. With reference to innumerate examples, it is absolutely true that ever since the usual suspects have been doing their utmost to undermine such legislation. It is clear (to those who choose to look) that a similar situation exists today and that the industry has evolved and become much more intelligent in how it communicates with (lies too) a given population. Which takes us nicely to another example of how *"the corporations"* buy the law, thus subjecting us all to the vicissitudes of the best democracy money can buy.

### The GRAS list

On New Year's Day 1958 the US Congress passed the Food Additives Amendment Act (FAAA). The act was supposed to ensure that all new substances developed by industry would be subject to thorough testing and review before being declared safe for human consumption. The onus was on the industry to test the safety of a given substance before it even got to the laboratories of the FDA. As far as I know, in 2017 this is still the case. Before 1958 the onus was on the FDA to challenge industry proclamations. The reader should be assured that the industry fought hard and dirty against such developments. For instance, the legal wrangling around the 1958 Delaney Clause [18] demonstrates how the industry views public health. This clause explicitly forbids adding any known carcinogens to any food. So what is any self-respecting criminal enterprise and its apologists within the scientific community to do? How about removing the clause instead of upholding the law? And guess what? That is exactly what happened, by 1996 [19] after several decades of off and on lobbying by the food industry, the Delany clause was removed from statute and consigned to the dumpster. As far as I know, there is no legislation anywhere in the legal framework of the entire world which seeks to establish links between cancer and chemicals in processed food. There was and now there isn't, Wonderful! An identical attitude is clear and present today, with perhaps Genetically Modified Organisms (GMO's) representing the most (but not only) ferocious aspect of the industry position. The US food industry has exploited one major loophole and likely many others not presented here. The loophole is a voluntary database called the Generally Recognised as Safe (GRAS) list. Since 1958 any component of *"big agriculture"* can declare any substance it likes as GRAS. They are then able to add it to food without telling the FDA it exists. Not that in its current form, the FDA particularly cares. The GRAS list is an open ended platform whereby the industry is able to exempt a substance from assessment if it can be classed as *"safe"* by qualified scientists who undertake rigorous testing of the chemicals in question. Any substance that has been used or added (to food) for *"a long period of time with no adverse effects on the population eating it"*, can be added to the GRAS list. Any substance that the industry deems as safe can be declared GRAS.

The industry can then see to it that any substance it chooses can be exempt from the *"formal food additive assessment process"* and this is exactly what happens. Potentially, any substance declared GRAS will find its way into the human chain. In 1980 the GRAS list contained 415 substances and about 100 new substances per year are added to the list. So the reader is invited to do the arithmetic. The reader will be pleased to know that things improve from here, well no, I was kidding they don't, they get worse. In 1997 a move by the industry lobbyists inside the US congress made it easier to get substances as *"GRAS notified"* as opposed to *"GRAS petitioned"*. In a petition, the FDA has final say on the safety of a given substance, but with a notification the final decision lays with the manufacturer. With a notification the industry decides on the safety of the substances it wants to incorporate into the diet. Here, all the industry has to do is notify the FDA of its decision. Since the turn of the 21st century, only a handful of new substances have been *"petitioned"*. A group called the Pew Charitable Trust carried out one of the few detailed reports which exist [20] in this area. This 2011 study asserts that up to *"several thousand"* substances are moving around inside the human food chain and none of them have been subject to any form of scientific testing or assessment. According to the study, this number is on top of the six to ten thousand additives which already exist in the food we eat or those which are used to make it. Chapter six outlines how aspartame gained regulatory approval in the early 1980's. It is now 2017 I wonder what else has been approved by similar nefarious means. I truly do dread to think what the future holds in this area, both in the US and the rest of the world. The literature is laden with examples of substances that are on the GRAS list, which should not be. Some of them are mentioned in the references in this chapter and the rest of this book. The reader does not need a degree in *"science"* to realise that ingesting hundreds of different synthetic chemicals on a regular basis is going to be *"unhealthy"*. For instance, the Butylated hydroxyl-anisole (BHA) mentioned in chapter two is on the GRAS list but is also a known carcinogen. It can also induce birth defects. The possibility of *"synergistic toxicity"* is also more than possible. Clearly, the more substances present in the food we eat, the more likely it is that such toxicological relationships will manifest themselves. The potential for even more *"cocktail effects"* will inevitably present themselves. These substances are added to increase profits. I do not see how any rational objective human being can come to a different conclusion. Such realities compel me to put *"food issues"* well and truly on the list called *"things to fix if we are to survive"* (See chapters two and three).

GRAS is one of those industry sponsored initiatives that is supposed to elicit trust from the population. We as people are supposed to be re-assured because each substance has been rigorously tested by highly qualified research scientists. To a certain extent, we have to keep our feet on the ground with these issues. Some substances on the GRAS and other approved safe to eat lists are going to be harmless and absolutely natural. Speaking personally, I have lost count of the times I have had to say to friends and campaigners, *"that is not exactly true"* or *"well, no that doesn't happen, this does"*. It may well be true that study X demonstrates that a small amount of a synthetic derivative from crude oil is not harmful to a given population of laboratory animals. However, what happens when such substances are eaten as part of a nominally *"Western diet"* over life time periods of time, by a very large population of human beings. Does this change the basic foundation of GRAS or the statutes behind e numbers? Would eating dozens of different additives on a daily basis, from the cradle to the grave, translate into a global epidemic of food allergies, food intolerances, cancers, obesity and its bedfellow diabetes? I would argue that it is more than a distinct possibility. I would also state that you don't need primary literature to come to such a conclusion. These and other questions are absolutely intertwined with recent food and additive controversies. The Southampton six is but one example. Or, as that freak across the pond, disguised as a human being, who is the president of the United States, his insane cabal of crooks and psychopaths, their moronic supporters and voting base like to believe, are these notions, the basis of a *"hoax"* perpetrated by external agencies that are out to bring down the United States? As with climate change, I know who I believe and it is isn't the self-serving thugs in suits who are turning our home in the cosmos into an atrophied wasteland in the name of profit.

## Where do E numbers come from?

The forerunner to the EU was a trading block known as the Common Market (EEC). This trading bloc didn't materialise out of some amorphous political nothingness. It came out of the destruction wreaked by World War Two. Huge regions of post second world war Europe and its people were traumatised and ravaged by the conflict. Many of its cities had been turned into rubble and millions of people were homeless. Millions in the East were left to the tender mercies of Josef Stalin's twisted interpretation of communism. Such are the consequences of not dealing with war mongering barbarians who run our affairs. To gain some idea of the scale of destruction the reader should peruse the current, system induced and intensifying catastrophes which have so devastated the Middle East, Northern and Western Africa as well as the global south. The EEC was born under the auspices of the Marshall Plan [21] which was set up to rebuild post war Europe as quickly as possible. The first tangible step toward what we now refer to as the EU took the form of the European Coal and Steel Community (ESCS [22]), which was established through the 1951 treaty of Paris. The list we refer to as e-numbers was developed throughout the 1950's. In 1962 the EEC created the mechanisms which allowed the first food colourants to be added to the emerging e number list. In 1964 preservatives were similarly added. In 1970 anti-oxidants followed suit. By 1974 emulsifiers, thickeners gelling agents and stabilisers were classified. The e number database is open ended.

Provided science can establish the safety of a given substance it can end up as an e number, which means you and I can and often do end up eating it. Organisation by e number establishes a framework for the identification of:

- Colourants E 100-199
- Preservatives E 200-299
- Anti-oxidants and acidity regulators E 300-399
- Thickeners, stabilisers and emulsifiers E 400-499
- Acidity regulators and anticaking agents E 500-599
- Flavour enhancers E 600-699
- Anti-biotics E 700-799
- Glazers and sweeteners E900-999
- Unclassified chemicals E 1000-1599

Most of the substances which fall into these categories are pre-fixed by a capital E. The E pre-fix means that the substance has been approved for use in the EU. The letter "E" indicates Europe and the unique number determines the name of the particular substance. Any derivatives or related compounds can be prefixed by an extra letter or number. For example, sorbitol [23] is denoted as E 420 (i) and sorbitol syrup is listed as E 420 (ii). Riboflavin [24] which is also called vitamin B2 is denoted by E 101 (i) and E 101 (ii) is riboflavin 5 phosphate. The latter form is likely to be made by the action of a genetically engineered bacterial microbe called Bacillus subtilis. From here it is possible to say how much of a particular substance can be safely (from the industries perspective) consumed and to what foods it can be legally added. The idea behind the prefix is to regulate the use of additives but not encourage it. Before the laws outlined in this chapter came into force food adulteration through to straight up poisoning was the issue to be dealt with. For instance, before the 1860 Food Adulteration Act (FAA) came into being:

- Tea was combined with soot to bulk it out.
- Flour was routinely mixed with ground up bones and/or

alum to increase its volume and whiteness.

- Calcium sulphate in the form of plaster of Paris, clay and sawdust was often mixed with dough before it was baked into bread. In the modern world, it is a key ingredient and additive for Tofu [25] and other soy bean based foods.
- Ammonium Carbonate [26] was used to mask the appearance and taste of spoiled flour. It can also be used as a leavening (rising) agent for some baked foods.
- Mixes of powdered dried pulses and rye flour were often substituted for real wholemeal flour.
- Unbelievably, for the 21st century, at any rate, mashed cow and calf brains were added to whipped cream to make it thicker.

Such were the practices employed to increase the volume of common foods. They happened with the express purpose of increasing profits for both manufacturers and vendors. In the Industrialised world, these extreme and criminal practices have been largely eradicated. The FAA is arguably one of several stepping stones to the regulations which are supposed to keep modern food fit for purpose. However, this does not mean everything is all rosy in modern intensive food production. This book clearly argues that the opposite holds true. The prolific, profit driven and unnecessary addition of thousands of substances have polluted the food which most of us eat on a daily basis. In the land of additives and food processing things are far from fresh, healthy, wholesome and nutritious. Plus the current situation is becoming even more precarious and deplorable on an almost daily basis. Theoretically, the approval process for all food additives is subject to rigorous testing and the pillars of objective science. In addition, the *"approved status"* is supposed to be monitored and if necessary reviewed. Yet, who the scientists are, the strength of the tests, why and how they are initiated is not made clear. Once again it is important to plainly state that many E numbers refer to substances that we are familiar with. In many cases, we have been using them for hundreds of years with no adverse impact at all. For instance, E 260 denotes acetic acid, (vinegar [27]). This very weak organic acid is used in pickling, one of our oldest and most effective methods of food preservation. The benefits of pickling are discussed in some detail in our well-thumbed *"farmhouse cookbook"*. The traditional cookbooks are light years ahead of the modern types. Any decent traditional farmhouse cookbook knocks the socks off most new cookbooks I have seen. Ours sits right next to the herb and spice rack, in the kitchen. Other beneficial additives or processing techniques include:

- Caramel (E 150 [28]), is a colouring agent that can easily be made at home by gently heating sugar. Large scale caramelisation is more complex than simply heating some sugar in a saucepan! Sadly, it is increasingly likely that the caramel used in food manufacture is derived from GM crops [29], most likely [30] corn or sugar beet.

- Baking powder or Bicarbonate of soda (sodium bicarbonate) E 500 [31] was developed in the late 19th century as a leavening agent for sourdough and spelt bread making. It is also used to make cakes, sponges and pastries. It is derived from a mineral called Trona [32] ($Na_2CO_3 \cdot NaHCO_3 \cdot 2H_2O$), the largest deposit in the world is in the US state of Wyoming. Alternatively, if you channel a mixture of $CO_2$ gas and ammonia through a solution of concentrated brine, lots of lovely crystals of baking powder will begin to precipitate out.

- The nitrites and nitrates (E249-252) – see below have been used as curing agents and preservatives for decades.

- The poly-saccharide pectin (E 440 [33]) a gelling and thickening agent. The synthetic variant is known as a methylated ester of galacturonic acid. It also belongs to the hydro-colloid family of chemicals mentioned in chapter one. The number E 440 is broken down into four different pectin containing compounds, i.e. E 440 (i-iv).

- Benzoic acid (E 210) was discovered in the 16th century and is found naturally in many plants and spices. For instance, plums, cranberries, cloves and cinnamon. It is slightly soluble in water and is an excellent food preservative. The most concentrated natural source of this substance is from the sap and gum of the Chinese Balsam Tree.

When last I checked all of the foods which contain Benzoic acid garner proven health benefits. As an additive, it prevents the growth of moulds and fungi. The case for using benzoic acid as a preservative is as strong now as it was when this particular property was discovered in the 19th century. However, as with all complex and inter-connected subjects, it just isn't that simple. With any substance that we come into contact with, especially on which we are eating, it is not unreasonable to ask where the benzoic acid used in food processing comes from. For example *"is it extracted from a natural source and then refined before being added to a given food"*? Or, *"is the benzoic acid produced from a laboratory in a chemical company which is connected to the manufacturer in question"*? In the body Benzoic acid plays a vital role in the elimination [34] of waste nitrogen. It also has utility in the treatment of certain genetic disorders. It is not the bad boy chemical [35] that some quarters have made it out to be. Having said that, some evidence suggests that benzoic acid and vitamin C (ascorbic acid) can react in the presence of light and heat to form benzene, which is a known carcinogen. However, we are all breathing in benzene and other carcinogens in the form of air pollutants. Plus, the inhaled concentrations are generally much higher than those found in the food we eat.

Nobody is saying that food processing is intrinsically a bad idea. One essential foundation of this book is to stress this very point. Equally, it is absolutely right to question what kinds of processes are going on and the need for the additives concerned. For instance historically, salting, smoking and drying were the main methods of stopping processed meats [36] from rotting. By far salting was the most common method, but it was not the action of common salt itself that did the preserving. The active substance was a compound called saltpetre,[37] or potassium nitrate ($KNO_3$). It is present naturally as a contaminant in rock salt (Sodium chloride or NaCl). Any meats treated with saltpetre were considered safe once the meat had turned a characteristic red colour. Until the mid-1920's saltpetre was the workhorse of meat preservation. It is still used in the 21st century and denoted by number E 252.[38] However, since 1925 just about every form of processed meat you can think of has been treated with nitrate and nitrite preservatives running from E 249 [39]-252. They gained approval by means of the DOA with regulatory responsibility being handed over to the FDA in 1927. Including saltpetre, all of these compounds function by changing the acidity and therefore environmental conditions of the food in question. What is perhaps less understood is that spoilage occurs because the food becomes a habitat for different microbes. One species of particular concern is known as *c. botulinum,* which belongs to the Clostridium bacterial family. As the reader can probably work out the bug causes the syndrome we know as botulism. The *c. botulinum* bacterium produces one of the most potent neurotoxins known to humanity. As far as human beings are concerned it is the most dangerous bacterium on the Earth. The microbe can and will kill, any person who becomes poisoned with it. The bug disrupts the nervous system by destroying nerve synapses. By doing so, the action of the neurotransmitters is also disrupted. If the bacteria are ingested [40] it will cause paralysis which begins with the facial area including the eyes. The paralysis spreads through the rest of the body before reaching the hands and feet. When the paralysis reaches the chest, the microbe stops the transmission of nerve impulses in the diaphragm and rib cage. You literally drown in a breathable atmosphere. Further symptoms include nausea, vomiting, double vision and slurred speech. Yes, indeed, botulism poisoning is a potentially fatal experience to avoid! So what does this have to with the nitrates and nitrites? Most microbes require the presence of oxygen to carry out their life process, c.botulinium does not. It is one of the relatively few microbes which live in oxygen deficient or completely anaerobic (oxygen free) environments.

By changing the environmental conditions for the microbes the meat became a less hospitable place for them. Saltpetre is a powerful oxidising agent which releases oxygen when it breaks down, this creates an environment which is toxic to c.botulinium. The Saltpetre prevents the sporulation (reproduction) of the microbe. Potassium nitrate is also essential for the manufacture of artificial fertilisers and gunpowder. Saltpetre is not as effective as the E numbers mentioned above. Although some outbreaks still occur, using the nitrate and nitrite additives has pretty much removed the c.botulinium microbe from the human food chain. Given that the consequences of botulism poisoning can be (and often are) fatal, it would seem that keeping c.botulinium out of the human food chain is a no-brainer. Weapons grade forms of this microbe are present in modern day biological weapons. A degraded (less toxic) variant of this microbe is the active substance employed for those who are disconnected enough from themselves to undergo cosmetic Botox treatment. The injection literally destroys the nerve endings in the skin which give us our characteristic features. The ability to express your emotions returns when the nerve endings begin to repair themselves. Clearly, repeated injections will do your peripheral nervous system long term damage. The US FDA granted approval for Botox treatment in 2002. Putting it directly, if you as an individual choose to undergo cosmetic Botox treatment you are injecting a proven neurotoxin into your body whose manufacture has probable links to the armaments industry.

**Perspectives on Food law in the modern world**

When you look at food processing in the modern world, standards have definitely improved, but the industry can still pretty much do what it wants. According to the references in excess of 10,000 individual chemicals are permitted for use in US processed foods. Similar numbers exist for the rest of the industrialised world. Although there may be differences between individual countries the broad strokes are essentially identical. Some of these substances are on the GRAS list whilst others are subject to more stringent legislation and safeguard. The modern food industry is acutely aware of how sensitive people are to any news concerning the safety of the foods we eat. It is also true if I were to pick a jar of *"brand X strawberry jam"* and send it off to a laboratory for analysis; the results would come back showing that levels of substances are well within legal limits. This reality is supposed to reassure us all that the food is safe and so we need not be concerned. Such is the essential foundation of what is called *"acceptable limits"*. There is not very much of a given substance in the food we eat and so there is no possibility of any harm if you eat the food in question. So just tuck in, enjoy, and don't worry about it. Hopefully, this book is going some way to establishing that things are much more complex and inter-related. What has become the doctrine of *"acceptable limits"* for substances, in our food (as well as the wider environment) can be traced back to the 16th century. A Swiss physician called Paracelsus [41] (1493-1541) whose real name was Theophrastus Aureolus Bombastus von Hohenheim is credited with a phrase *"the dose maketh the poison"*. A statement which forms the basis of modern toxicology, the branch of science concerned with the study of toxins and their effects. Paracelsus was stating that for a given substance a small amount will not cause harm. Conversely, if enough of any substance is ingested it will cause harm by one mechanism or another. The trick is to establish at what concentration the substance starts to elicit harm, i.e. its toxicological effect. The effects of a toxin are one way to knock the organ systems of any organism out of balance. When the body is working as it should it is said to be operating within *"homeostatic"* [42] limits. The body and its organ systems are in balance with each other. Ingesting too much of any substance will upset the homeostatic balance of our metabolism and some toxic effect or consequence will express itself. For example, drinking too much water causes the fluid membrane which surrounds the brain to expand causing haemorrhaging. However, a person would need to ingest many tens of litres of water at one sitting for such a toxic response to occur. Conversely, the toxicity of the botulism microbe is measured in nano-grams. One nanogram is one billionth of a gram. In the 16th century most of the substances mentioned in this book simply did not exist, likely they would not have even been thought possible to exist. At this time science was just beginning to take its first journeys into the world of the microbes. Had Paracelsus known of such substances and organisms, likely, he would have cause to rethink his whole understanding of dose and poison. Life in the 16th century was not in any way countryside chocolate box living. It was the opposite of any romantic notions you may have. However, the diet was not laden with the additives that permeate the modern human food chain. Paracelsus did not slake his thirst with soft drinks laden with artificial sweeteners or excessive amounts of refined sugar. He would not sit down to a hearty ready meal for one because it was convenient. He didn't go to the local take away because there was no other option and he didn't visit food outlets that contained absolutely no fresh fruit or vegetables. Although I'm sure the streets of 16th century Switzerland had a lot to be desired Paracelsus was not exposed to industrial, traffic or urban pollution to anything like the degree most of us are today. The in(f)ternal combustion engine did not exist and coal, wood and to a lesser extent whale oil were the principal energy sources in 16th century Europe. There was exposure to toxic substances and I'm not saying otherwise. However, the levels and diversity of toxins were significantly less than it is in the 21st century. It is these toxins, pesticides, industrial chemicals and food additives that are studied and evaluated in modern food laboratories. The results of the analysis are then used to establish the degree of toxicity set against notions of acceptable limits and substantial equivalence.

The notion of *"acceptable limits"* is not a mentality unique to the processed food industry; it permeates throughout modern manufacturing and industry. For instance, in the mid-1990's the first foods grown from genetically engineered seeds were introduced with no warning or real discussion. The GM industry and the wider food industry have become exceptionally good at deflecting any concerns about their activities. One technique is to take a position called *"substantial equivalence"* (detailed in the *"Introducing GMO's"* book). The term exists on the US FDA website and became *"statute"* in the early 1980's. Successive governments (and the regulatory authorities behind them), in the EU and the Far East, have taken a similar line. Substantial equivalence means that natural, engineered and synthetic copies are *"substantially equivalent"* to each other. There is no need for extra regulation because the *"natural"* and *"synthetic"* are identical. An acceptable limit exists for the consumption of the synthetic form. All of the chemical substances and genetically engineered organisms in existence are safe and therefore not problematic. The food industry is not alone in defending its use of artificial substances or production processes which generate suspicion and therefore question. Every industry on the planet defends its corner with exactly the same sort of nonsense. The consequences of this level of acceptance are clear and present to those of us who choose to look and campaign against it. An opposite position called the *"precautionary principle"* [43] is woefully absent. It is at best an afterthought in the minds of those who regulate and operate within the food industry. With a precautionary approach the focus is on assessing whether the substance is needed in the first place, often it isn't. Hopefully, this book is making clear that most modern additives only exist for the benefit of the food industry itself. With the precautionary principle, the slightest hint of damage to people or planet spurs on the development of ever more safer substances for a given process. This is an attitude which should be applied in all industries and human endeavours. Sadly, it isn't and the consequences are there at local, regional, national, international and global level for everyone to observe. During the course of the research carried out on food processing I have seen no evidence that the manufacturers are remotely interested in removing as many additives as possible from their products, conversely, the opposite appears to be occurring. This is as true of intensive food production and food processing as it is with GMO's. The activities and practices which occur in the food processing industry appear for all intents and purposes to be unregulated. Having stated the obvious, the food [44] and related industries are in possession of a metaphorical self-preservation gene and will act to remove any substances which are clearly or potentially toxic. Be assured that the removal [45] of such compounds is not occurring out of any concern for the health of you, yours or the planet on which you live. It occurs because they can do without the hassle or the cost such hassle can generate. There is no guarantee that any replacement compounds are going to be any different. In a world which is awash with thousands of individual human made compounds which are merrily cycling their way through the entire Earth and every living organism upon it, such developments are a moot point.

As for the scientists and food engineers in the employ of the industry I am absolutely sure they believe in what they are doing and that it is for the betterment of all. Exactly the same can be said for the genetic engineers who are employed by the biotechnology and life science companies. However, any social, geo-political, economic and environmental context in which the products of their research will be applied is completely missing from their collective thought process. In that world, if the science demonstrates that the substance in question is safe and the science is sound and peer reviewed then there is not supposed to be a problem. From this position, those of us who ask questions on these subjects are seen as the problem and not the existence of the subject itself. Even worse institutions and individuals who view other ways of seeing the world as somehow *"unscientific"* tend to follow a similar trajectory. I am in no way suggesting that evidence should be substituted for conjecture (or vice versa), quite the opposite. I am imparting and in the strongest possible terms, that *"science"* in and of itself is not always enough, especially when it is applied to public health, the environment, and food additives. These highly skilled individuals are so hopelessly inert when it comes to the types of questions posed by this kind of writing that they cannot cope, don't answer pertinent points and resort to personal attack. Consequently, the proclivity to deny, project, distract and deflect and obstruct at every opportunity is clear and present. Well, that is what happens to me, maybe it's my exposition! Personally, I'm sick of it, I left that behaviour behind in the school playground, or I thought I had. Perhaps the reader would like to ask the people in their lives the same sort of questions and keep doing so, to test the hypothesis? Such people are absolutely science-centric, in that the *"science"* supersedes all other concerns. Including your innate right to act rationally and decide for yourself what is good to eat. Even in today's increasingly autocratic and unhinged world, you do have the right to say *"No,"* even if a substance is not in scientific terms toxic. In a similar vein I have lost patience with meaningless platitudes of acceptance, this belter being one of my favourites, *"but billions of meals have been cooked with GM ingredients"*. After I have said, *"I don't want to eat it and would rather eat food produced from organic and/or permaculture systems"*. Such perspectives are consistently ignored by those agencies and individuals who operate solely on scientific terms. And yes Golden Rice and Vitamin A bananas (as but two examples) I am looking at you. How about rectifying the systemic reasons as to why so many people on Planet Earth in the 21st century are wondering where their next meal is coming from? Chapter six demonstrates how many substances gain their approval, how the construct which develops them operates and most importantly what it thinks of you. All points considered I would argue that the notion of a right to say no morphs directly into a responsibility.

In that world, the science itself is *"value free"*, meaning it is totally separate from the real world in which it is applied. Clearly, if we are talking about additives and GMO's such a position is absolutely and completely oxymoronic. More severely, it represents an abdication of responsibility which is tantamount to deliberate abuse of science, people and the planet which supports us all. These scientists consider those of us who are concerned about additives, food production and/or opposed to GMO's as being *"stupid and anti-science"*. For instance, on a recent Programme presented by Professor Brian Cox the question *"what do you think of those who are opposed to GMO's?"* was posed to a GM research scientist in the employ of the biotechnology industry. His response was, and I quote directly, *"they are stupid people to the point of criminality because they are holding back the course of objective reasoned and well directed genetic engineering"*. To scientists and researchers who think and say such things, the rest of us, are not living in the real world. Our opposition to what is being done (to the species, the planet and every living organism on it) in general and GMO's, in particular, is not something to be acknowledged or respected. Our questions and concerns are a resistance to the progress of science and the scientific method. The resistance and questioning is to be ground down or circumvented by any means necessary. Sadly, I have to say that such people and the industry which pays their wages have been very successful in this department. A more succinct way to present the strategy is to frame it under the heading *"lobbying"* and it's equally unpleasant cousin *"bribery"*. Of late with such people my scientific gloves have come off and been discarded for good. The flim-flam the gloves used to represent no longer exists. The people I speak of are not interested in any meaningful discourse on these subjects. They truly will say and do anything except look in the mirror and admit their own culpability. Collectively, they are supine, obsequious, deluded and cowardly ideologues who sold themselves out a long time ago. Speaking personally, such people can go and fuck themselves, ideally in prison where they belong. Thankfully, such protagonists are not in the majority that they think they are and their research is not as water tight as they like to pretend it is. Like all criminals these people are engaged in two fundamental activities, one is *"pretending"* and the other is *"lying"*. And make no mistake they are exceptionally good at both, so much so they believe their own delusions. Chapter six on the regulatory framework which led to aspartame approval is only one example of such activity. They also miss the overriding point and essence of the precautionary principle. If the additives themselves were much less present then avoiding them would be a moot point because they would not exist in the quantities or combinations that they currently do.

All of this loops straight back to chapter three. We are looking at risk avoidance, so if you don't want the risk of developing any potential problems, avoid these foods and the substances they contain wherever you can. It really is that simple. Food additives and processing is a deeply controversial issue. Yet, it is a controversy rooted in the organisation of human society. It is not a controversy [46] of my making or of anyone who is concerned about how food issues fit into questions concerning how the world is organised. The whole issue is a consequence of capitalisms own making, so it is not my fault or that of anyone else who challenges that system. Putting it bluntly:

- The controversy is not going to end whilst thousands of substances are routinely added with little or no scrutiny to the food we eat.
- The controversy is not going to end solely because the science is stated as being sound.
- The controversy is not going to end while far too many professional people refuse to look in the mirror.
- The controversy will not end whilst far too many scientists

169

do not speak out against that which is so manifestly wrong.

- The controversy will not end whilst corporate sponsored science is the norm and not the exception.
- The controversy will not end while the Western diet exists and all other forms of food production are subsumed on the altar of profit.
- The controversy will not end whilst far too many people see the western diet as the norm.
- The controversy will not end while big agriculture exists.

The controversy **WILL** end when agriculture and food production is carried out so that everybody on the planet has access to healthy nutritious food. The controversy **WILL** end when said food is affordable and accessible to all. The controversy **WILL** end when agriculture is seen as a component of nature and biodiversity and not in conflict with it. The controversy **WILL** end when food processing exists solely for the reasons that human beings started it carrying out in the first place. The controversy **WILL** end when agriculture is carried out for the benefit of all. The controversy **WILL** end when agriculture is hardwired into human organisation as part of a genuinely sustainable future for all. And that boys and girls is the fundamental point of this book. The next chapter provides a text book example of exactly what I am driving at; sadly it is not an isolated case.

# Chapter Six: Aspartame – An Overview Demonstrating How Not To Regulate

Perhaps the most obvious example of what is so wrong with the Western diet is the plastic bottles and aluminium cans which contain soft drinks. There are plenty of *"political"* and *"environmental"* reasons to remove such beverages from your diet. Collectively, they ought to be added to the examples which make up chapter three. The same can be said of the fare on offer from the KFC's, Burger Kings and McDonald's of this world. Leaving all other points aside the burgers are not burgers, the chicken is not chicken and the salads are not salads. The food on offer from such outlets is called junk food for a reason. It has absolutely no nutritional value what so ever and is loaded to the max with substances that ought not to be ingested by any organism alive or any that has ever lived since the time of the Archean [1]. This geologic time period is delimited by the dating of the oldest known rocks on the Earth; they are some 3.8 Billion years old. The first life on Earth is known to have appeared some 3.6 billion years ago, the first fossils which prove the existence of life are some 3.2 billion years old. Having said that, research published in September 2017, puts the earliest known life even further back into deep time. The Archean ended approximately 2.5 billion years ago, with the emergence of Eukaryotes. The first single celled organisms which also contained a nucleus. I like to think such organisms ignore big mac or whopper burgers, so I choose not to eat them either! Fast food is not by any definition food and that alone is reason enough to avoid it. The soft drinks available from the fast food outlets are no different. A Soft drink is really a catch all term which means any non-alcoholic beverage. This chapter will only be looking at fizzy drinks including energy and fitness drinks. Referring back to chapter three, a guaranteed method for reducing the health impacts of processed foods is to avoid fizzy carbonated drinks where ever possible. Leaving aside the sound ethical, moral and political reasons to avoid certain brands of soft drink, the reasoning is that they have no nutritional value whatsoever. In my experience, they do not even slake your thirst, even when they are ice cold. Having said that, none of us are perfect and I am no exception. Upon the death of Lemmy from Motorhead on December 28th 2015, my girlfriend and I certainly imbibed of his favourite beverage (Jack Daniels and Coca-Cola) by way of saying goodbye. We even had the hangover to prove it! The figures for soft drink consumption are pretty stark. For example, according to the Mercola website (listed below) the average American consumes some 700 cans of various fizzy drinks every year, so we can call it two cans a day. An article[2] in TIME magazine translates this number into about 165 litres per person per year. However, I was surprised to discover that Mexicans consume more fizzy drinks per capita than any other people on Earth. The figure exceeds the US per capita number by some 40%. Unsurprisingly, the nation has one of the highest obesity and diabetes rates on Earth. Other peoples are not so enamoured with fizzy drinks. In South Korea, the figure is somewhere near 27 litres per person. Here in Europe, we drink on average about half the US amount. Unsurprisingly the UK consumes more per year than our continental peers. As for Aspartame (ASP) in soft drinks, it may be approaching end game. For instance, The Pepsi Cola Company announced [3] in 2015 [4] that it was removing ASP from diet Pepsi, for the US part of its operations [5]. From here the glaringly obvious question poses itself, "*well, if it (ASP) is no longer in US Pepsi, why is it present here?*" Well, the substitution of ASP for a mix of sucralose [6] and acesulfame potassium (Ace-K) [7] is certainly not occurring because of any concern that Pepsi has for our collective health. Ace-K has identical sweetening properties to ASP but is not metabolised, hence the substitution. However, ace-k is still an artificial sweetener with a dubious regulatory track record. A record which stretches back into the early 1970's and in that sense is just as problematic as ASP. Acesulfame potassium is denoted as E 950 [8] and has the formula $C_4H_4KNO_4S$. The compound has been routinely used since it was approved in 1988. It is marketed under trade names including Sunnet and sweet one and manufactured [9] by the usual giant food conglomerates, or the subsidiaries they have set up or brought out. In addition, one of the solvents (methylene chloride / di-chloro-methane [10]) used to produce Ace-K is a potential occupational carcinogen. Given that I used this substance in varying concentrations throughout my time at university, I was somewhat perturbed to assimilate that particular nugget of information. This compound is a volatile and powerful organic solvent used by industries ranging from paint and metal stripping to pharmaceuticals as well as sweetener manufacturer. If I were writing about Ace-K I would find similar issues as those connected to ASP. Ace-K could also have had its own section in chapter seven. Plus, were it as well-known and studied as ASP, it could have been the subject of this chapter. The reader can assume it has equivalent metabolic problems as the sweeteners outlined in chapter seven. From a dietary perspective the switch from ASP to Ace-K will likely represent a frying pan to fire jump or deck chair movement on the sinking Titanic. Chapter seven also imparts that another replacement chemical for ASP, a substance called neotame, is merely a deck chair on the Titanic movement. The rest of this chapter focuses on ASP and its approval for human consumption. The only reason soft drinks are mentioned is because so many of them contain ASP. Having said that the reader should be absolutely clear that ASP and other artificial sweeteners (see chapter seven) are found in sweets, desserts, diet products and they are used as table top sweeteners. These substances are also present in some medicines. ASP has been deemed safe for human consumption in the US since 1981 and has had equivalent [11] status in the UK and EU since 1994. In the EU ASP is designated by the number E 951 [12]. At time of writing ASP has been approved safe for human consumption in approximately 90 countries.

In the interests of getting the science right, it has to be stated that for most of us, much of the hyperbole surrounding ASP is just that. However, there are clear and present health risks and serious questions remain concerning the approval process. ASP is absolutely one of the many thousands of additives which simply should not be present in the food most people on planet Earth eat on a daily basis. That is, assuming there is enough to eat in the first place. A crucially important point to make emphatically clear is that ASP is not eaten in isolation from the other artificial sweeteners. It is eaten as one synthetic substance in combination with the additives present in processed food. The science behind the ASP approval process was anything but objective and independent. By definition, it cannot be considered as *"good science"*. Should a person experience any negative symptoms from ingesting ASP, the industry position succinctly blames the individual. That is eating amounts outside of their stated *"acceptable limits"*, from this perspective any health impacts are our responsibility. The current (2017) Acceptable Daily Intake for ASP is 40mg/kg of food. According to the manufacturers themselves, one can of common diet soft drink more than exceeds [13] this amount. In some cases by over three times, if this is the lay of the land something is not right. Speaking personally I cannot be assured of the safety of any processed food when such obvious contradictions present themselves. As with GMO's and the wider processed food industry, the notion of not making such chemicals (or novel organisms) in the first place is entirely missing from the narrative. We shall be returning to the connections between ASP and GMO's in due course. For now, it is sufficient to state that ASP is derived from a genetically engineered form of E.coli bacteria. This particular strain has been engineered [14] to produce huge quantities of phenylalanine and aspartic acid. The E.coli is cultured and fermented for several days and the raw materials (the amino acids) collected. Amino acids produced in this way are important precursor compounds for the processed food industry.

In the world of objective science (and basic humanity) a whole corpus of knowledge and research augments the case that consuming ASP can and frequently does elicit the symptoms presented below. Perhaps this is why ASP is banned in Japan and *"officially discouraged"* in China. Perhaps this is why there are so many investigations and pushes for outright bans happening all over the world. Hundreds of primary scientific papers concerning the toxicity (or not) of ASP have been peer reviewed and published. Clearly, claim and counter claim permeate through the whole controversy. As the final paragraph in chapter five makes incisively clear, such controversies are not of my or anyone else's making. They are a direct result of decisions taken by the profiteering psychopaths and enemies of humanity who run things. I am willing to bet that those responsible care not a jot for the consequences of their actions. Having said that, it is fiendishly difficult to state absolutely that exposure to any individual substance will definitely cause adverse health impacts in animal populations, including human beings. Any reported health impacts cannot generally be placed at the door of a single substance and that goes for ASP too. Any issues forthcoming need to be viewed as one component of a wider analysis, critique or even attack on the modern food industry. To paraphrase Paracelsus (see chapter five) in modern prose, there is no such thing as a completely safe compound, just differing degrees of toxicity. In any organism, if levels of any substance become too high it will express some form of toxicity. It's all about the quantity and source of substances being ingested by the individual. As such, there is no such thing as a completely safe substance. Outside of industry circles, the potential [15] health impacts of ASP are well documented and understood. Conversely, on the other side of the coin hundreds of millions of people regularly consume foods and drinks which contain ASP. Along with ingesting other artificial sweeteners no adverse health impacts are reported. So, we can legitimately ask who is right. As a believer in the precautionary principle, I choose to remove such considerations from my own life and food choices. And I do that by not consuming any foods which contain ASP or indeed any artificial sweeteners (see chapter seven) of any kind whatsoever. Leaving such personal choices aside three obvious questions beg themselves right in front of us:

- What is Aspartame?
- How did it gain approval?
- Should we be concerned?

So, here we are then on the train to the land of ASP, its regulation and consequences thereof, all aboard? Choo, Choo and we're off........

## What is Aspartame?

ASP is a wholly synthetic compound. It is not found anywhere in the natural world. Along with all the other artificial sweeteners and human made food additives, it is an absolutely novel substance. It is approximately 200 times sweeter than white refined table sugar (sucrose) but contains only between 1 and 4 percent of the calorific value. According to the literature ASP was discovered completely by accident. Aside from the next generation of molecules, in the world of artificial sweeteners, accidental discoveries are the norm. The dubious credit for the discovery of ASP goes to a scientist called Jim Schlatter. The discovery of ASP is rooted in research which was looking to improve treatment for gastric ulcers. The research was funded by a pharmaceutical company called G D Searle [16], who are now part of the obscenely bloated pharmaceutical conglomerate Pfizer. [17] In 1965, so the story goes, as different compounds were discovered, Mr Schlatter accidentally tasted one of them. He was, so the story goes, blown away by the intensely sweet taste caused by a minute quantity of the white solid that became known as ASP. The full chemical name for ASP [18] is N-(L-α-Aspartyl)-L-phenylalanine, 1-methyl ester, the formula is

$C_{14}H_{18}N_2O_5$. From a chemical point of view, ASP is not a particularly complex molecule. By mass it is made up of:

- 40% Aspartic Acid [19]
- 50% Phenylalanine
- 10% Methanol / Methyl Ester

As an essential amino acid phenylalanine can only be obtained from proteins in the diet. Aspartic acid is a non-essential amino acid meaning it can be manufactured by the body. The methyl ester forms when methanol chemically bonds with phenylalanine. It is this ester bond which gives ASP its intensely sweet taste. Esters are discussed in the Food Conspiracy book and are mentioned in chapter one. ASP has been present in the human food chain since 1974 when it was first approved as a dry food additive. A key, if not the key, driver to the approval was the approximately 100 papers submitted by GD Searle to the FDA during 1973. Fast forward through the several decades to 2017 and ASP is found in processed [20] food products [21] pretty much everywhere. ASP is present in:

- Alcohol-free beer and cider
- Desserts
- Fruit juices made from concentrate
- Preserved and tinned fruits
- Jams and marmalades
- Spreads, low-fat spreads and butter substitutes
- Diet and regular soft drinks
- Milk drinks and ice cream
- Sweets and chocolates
- Prescription and non-prescription medicines
- Cordials and squashes
- Condiments, sauces and pastes

The chances are if the label says *"no added sugar"*, *"diet"*, *"max"*, *"sugar-free"* or *"light"* then that particular product has in the past or is still likely to contain [22] ASP. Trade names for ASP include NutraSweet, Canderel, NutraTaste, Benevia, Amino Sweet, equal, spoonful and equal measure.

## Aspartame Metabolism

When a person digests ASP it is rapidly broken down into its constituent molecules, (the two amino acids and the methyl ester). It takes seconds for the methyl ester bond to be broken. When the bond breaks methanol [23] ($CH_3OH$) is liberated. Methanol is the first substance in the alcohol family of organic compounds. The ethanol most of us consume in our various favourite tipples is the second compound in the series. However, methanol (methylated spirit or wood alcohol) is much more toxic [24] than ethanol. The ester bond in ASP is broken down in the small intestine. The methanol is then absorbed into the blood stream and transported to the liver. There it is converted to formaldehyde and then formic acid [25] (HCOOH). This is a well understood metabolic pathway and the liver is well adapted to deal with normal dietary i.e. non-toxic levels of methanol. However, it is the formic acid which causes the truly horrific consequences of methanol poisoning. The reader must not form the impression that consuming a diet drink is the equivalent to drinking a bottle of methylated spirits because it isn't. You are not going to go blind if you drink a can of diet artificially sweetened carbonated water. However, the metabolic process which converts the methanol is identical in both instances. And it is here that one of the myths of ASP presents itself. It simply is not true that drinking fizzy drinks (or any other dietary source) which contain ASP, will make a person go blind. You would need to ingest handfuls of pure ASP at one sitting for that to happen. The main concern around ASP centres on the role of its metabolites (break down products) in the symptoms [26] indicated below. Having made this point clear, methanol can have negative impacts on sensitive individuals in some circumstances.

Methanol can interact with a neurotransmitter [27] called dopamine [28] and from there upset the delicate *"pleasure-reward cycle"* (see chapter seven) which can lead to addiction in susceptible individuals. Dopamine is also a precursor chemical to adrenaline and can affect the efficacy of the *"fight or flight response"*. The science speaks for itself a peer reviewed [29] journal called "Aspartame, Methanol and Public Health" presented research which concludes *"When diet sodas and soft drinks, sweetened with aspartame, are used to replace fluid loss during exercise and physical exertion in hot climates, the intake of methanol can exceed 250 mg/day or 32 times the Environmental Protection Agency's recommended limit of consumption for this cumulative poison."* Elevated levels of phenylalanine (see below) are known to compromise the manufacture of dopamine and serotonin. The neurotransmitters have many functions and are absolutely essential for our mental health. They promote cognisance, mental agility, memory as well as regulating our temperament. Higher levels of phenylalanine can upset the transport of amino acids across the blood brain boundary and have been associated with the onset of epilepsy [30]. A key problem with aspartame metabolism does not focus on methanol, rather, the quantities of amino acid ingested. When ASP is digested the phenylalanine and aspartic acid are liberated. In an omnivorous diet, the aspartic acid and phenylalanine quotient is very roughly about 5% of the total amino acid ingested. There is no concern if you are ingesting them in situ and in balance with other essential nutrients. The ratio of amino acids found in aspartame simply does not occur in either animal or plant proteins. Consequently, the body has more metabolic work to do as compared to the same substances found in natural protein sources. It is this difference which potentially makes aspartame an excitotoxin. An Excitotoxin is any amino acid which causes over stimulation of nerve cells. In this state, hence the term excitotoxin, the human nervous system transmits impulses much more rapidly than they otherwise would. In affected cells, the end result is their self-termination (cellular apoptosis). ASP has also been implicated in a reported and well established increase in the numbers [31] of brain tumours [32] across the western world. Any kind of supposition which links any synthetic substance to adverse effects on human health is bound to invite controversy. Again I have to say I accept no responsibility for such controversies. I blame the manufacturers, their scientific stooges and the system they are part of, end of story! Research in this area has been progressing since before ASP was even approved. For example, in 1996 researchers from Kings College in London collated findings from 166 peer reviewed studies concerning the impact of ASP. According to the lead author (Dr Ralph G Walton), there were 74 studies commissioned by the food industry and none of them found any negative impacts. Yet, 84 of the remaining 92 found some sort of adverse effect. On this basis alone I would argue that consuming ASP just isn't worth the risk. And so I present another example of why the advice presented in chapter three really ought to be followed for ASP. I also impart this point of view from a climate perspective. It appears that Dr Walton does not believe that human activity is inducing climate change. Now, I believe based on overwhelming evidence, on a solid understanding of Earth, environmental and a system science perspective that, human induced climate change is a mass extinction level reality of cataclysmic proportions. Climate change has been in the past and there is absolutely every reason that it will be again. It is just that far too many people just don't seem to realise or more worryingly care. I agree with Dr Walton's position on ASP, but not with his view on climate change. Such is the dynamic world of the social and environmental sciences; truly there is no one size fits all.

Anyway back to ASP! In 1996 the US Congress was told in absolute crystal clear language by a chief toxicologist from the USFDA called Dr Adrian Gross (now deceased) that *"without a shadow of a doubt aspartame can cause brain tumours and brain cancer"*. To date (August 2017) the FDA has not reviewed the status of this ubiquitous sweetener and as far as I can ascertain has no intention [33] of doing so. The reticence on the part of the FDA is perhaps understandable (if completely immoral) when we factor in the Delaney amendment, see chapter five. This provision (which was removed from US law in 1996) explicitly prohibits the addition of any known carcinogen (a substance which causes cancer [34]) to the human or animal food chain. The inference from such shenanigans should be obvious. If you can't crush or rubbish dissent on an issue, simply remove the legal basis for expressing it. Scientists are by the nature of their profession objective and generally try not to let *"emotion"* get in the way of results. This is not saying that they don't care, just that the evidence or *"what the results and data tell us"* takes precedence over what our opinion on a given issue is. This is what scientists mean when they say their work is value free. There is no judgement to be made or opinion to be had and if the science is robust, objective and conclusions match results. Having a value free perspective is all well and good if we are settling a debate on the composition of a distant star or deciding on a given aspect of evolutionary theory. However, the notion that science is *"value free"* when it is applied to the world in which we live, where the application has consequences, quickly disintegrates. Well, it does if you understand the relationship between action and reaction, the difference between cause and consequence. Value free judgements collapse if you know how to question, the state of things, what is being done (and has been done) in the world today and throughout our history. So, for example, when a scientist (Dr Gross) who is in the employ of a government agency expresses *"shock"* at an inexplicable spike in the incidence of brain and other tumours in the US population and other qualified professionals, in this frame, Dr. Russel Blaylock follow suit, we as members of the public ought to be concerned. Any person who does not express concern about such matters is a prime candidate for the next edition of the Darwin Awards. According to Dr Blaylock (who has written several books on this subject) *"They (the sweetener industry) all realized that they couldn't answer my arguments. So they left me alone. They're afraid that if it comes to a big standoff between me and them, they're going to lose. What they're doing is the old ploy of just ignoring and hoping it will go away. They put pressure on magazines, journals and newspapers not to interview me. They are trying to keep me in the shadows where they hope most people don't hear anything I have to say. It only works for so long."* As with a page called *"the trouble maker"* 35 in the UK based hard and revolutionary left (as opposed to the centre/ reformist left) socialist worker, if what is being said is untrue, why don't the accused go after the accuser? The reason is obvious and dovetails exactly with the above quote from Dr Blaylock. As a sensible rational person, I happen to believe in the precautionary principle. So, if I can avoid damage to my health or person, even if the risk is remote, then I will. In the case of impacts on the human nervous system, we are discussing damage which is irreversible. If you will excuse the pun, from a neurological perspective avoiding ASP is a no brainer. The neurological impact of artificial sweeteners is outlined in chapter seven.

ASP has a wonderfully dysfunctional honour. It is the most studied artificial sweetener in existence. As such it represents yet another long running industry created controversy. If it had never been developed and marketed I would not be writing this chapter. A point which applies to most of the substances mentioned in this book. We only know the degree of study concerning ASP because of a demand in 1995 under the US equivalent of the Freedom of Information act. Five years before the 21st-century began; the FDA was compelled to make public the complete list of symptoms reported by over 10,000 individuals. According to the literature, the FDA approached the Atlanta Centre for Disease Control, who reviewed the first 650 complaints. Various sources cite the figure of 10,000 as representing over 75% of **ALL** complaints about food additives to the FDA. If this is true since the creation of the FDA in 1906 most complaints have been down to one synthetic compound. On top of that, they have been levied only since the mid 1970's.

Now, if that is not a clear cut example of the imbalance which permeates throughout our lives in the western world, I don't know what is. There is a 16-year lapse between the discovery of ASP and its approval. The timeline of events surrounding this accidental compound is as shocking as it is unsurprising. As of September 2017, ASP is found in thousands of individual processed foods, but most is ingested via diet fizzy drinks. An entrenched belief exists in that people believe ASP in particular and sweeteners, in general, will help you lose weight. Given the advertising and promotion of them, this is hardly surprising. The reasoning is simply that their calorific value is practically zero. Chapter seven will outline how this position is becoming progressively more untenable [36].

## Aspartame, Phenylketonuria (PKU) and Risk Assessment

Over the years 1974 to 1981 ASP was approved for use as a dry additive only. In 1981 ASP became approved for use as a general purpose sweetener. Even in the mid 1970's serious [37] questions were asked over ASP and the scientific basis for its status as being *"safe for human consumption"*. As with GMO's and other additives, the question as to whether or not we want to eat it in the first place was deliberately conspicuous in its absence. The chances are that you and your family regularly ingest it. If you imbibe of diet fizzy drinks and use artificial sweeteners, it is almost certain that ASP is regularly broken down by your metabolism. Ever since approval was facilitated by the collusion of Donald Rumsfeld and Arthur Hayes (see below), ASP was on track for being the subject of more complaint to the FDA than any other additive. ASP is known to interact with:

- Anti-depressants
- Some neurotransmitters
- Coumadin (brand name warfarin) an anti-coagulant or blood thinning molecule
- Individual Hormones and the endocrine (hormonal)

system
- Various Cardiac medications
- Vaccines

It should not surprise anyone to see why so many complaints are associated with this artificial substance. Elevated levels of blood phenylalanine is a critical factor for the approximate one in ten thousand individuals who have inherited phenylketonuria (PKU) [38]. Screening for PKU is standard across the western world. The screening is necessary because people with PKU cannot metabolise phenylalanine. For a person with PKU phenylalanine is effectively a poison. If it builds up in the body brain damage and other serious conditions are the result. A person with PKU is missing an enzyme called phenylalanine hydroxylase [39] (PAH). Enzymes are proteins which catalyse the rate of specific biochemical reactions. The production of enzymes is coded for by DNA. PAH converts phenylalanine into tyrosine (another amino acid) which is then converted into the skin pigment melanin. With individuals who have PKU, the conversion doesn't happen and phenylalanine starts accumulating in the circulatory system. Consequently, [40] people with PKU have lighter skin and hair colour than those whose DNA can code for manufacturing the PAH enzyme. People with PKU may have albino like characteristics but the two conditions are completely different. In younger children, the build-up of phenylalanine causes brain damage. The impact is so severe that mental retardation is inevitable if the accumulation is not stopped. Explaining why screening for PKU is mandatory, at least in the industrialised world. I wonder how many lives have been ruined because equivalent measures do not exist in the wider world. If too much phenylalanine is present then a PKU diagnosis is likely. PKU is not necessarily a life threatening condition but people who have been diagnosed need to monitor their diet [41] throughout their lives. A person with PKU has to avoid or precisely regulate their consumption of any high protein foods including many staples of a plant based diet. If PKU has been diagnosed the child needs to avoid high protein foods. The metabolism of ASP explains why any food or drink which contains it must be labelled. However, if the food manufacturers and industry were genuinely concerned about our health they would not be opposed to mandatory labelling for all the additives found in the food we eat. And we wouldn't need to petition them or compel them to do so, it would just happen. As a corollary, you could then be forgiven for asking *"why the additives are there in the first place?"* Exactly the same questions hold in any discussions on GMO's and their impact on human health and the environment.

According to doctors, toxicologists and health professional's aspartame causes and/or is implicated in conditions including but not limited to:

- Headache and migraine
- Loss of memory and vision
- Fits and seizures
- Coma
- Birth defects
- Autoimmune diseases
- Brain and neural [42] cancer
- Neurotoxicity to the brain, spinal cord and peripheral nervous system
- Impaired hearing

As written previously there is plenty of hyperbole and myth surrounding ASP. For example, talk of epidemics is exactly that, talk and unfounded assertion. However, this does not mean that ASP is safe or that it (and other compounds) should be in the food we eat. Just in case you needed any more reason to be cautious aspartame can intensify or even worse mimic symptoms of diseases or conditions including:

- Multiple Sclerosis
- Fibromyalgia [43] (a chronic rheumatoid disease)
- Lupus (an auto immune disease)

- ADD/ADHD
- Diabetes
- Alzheimer's [44]
- Chronic fatigue / ME
- Depression

Unsurprisingly, the science behind all of this is skewed and the results are conflicting. I say the controversy is entirely the fault of G.D Searle and those who allowed it to be approved. Those who see no issue with ASP believe (or publicly state) that the ASP controversy is a non-issue with no scientific merit. Such a position ignores the social and political context in which ASP and other additives are, developed, applied, consumed and promoted. It also ignores the reality that it is not uncommon for people who have none of these syndromes to experience them after long term consumption of ASP. The sweetener is not triggering a latent syndrome but is eliciting them in people who have no history of them. It may well be due to a cocktail effect of ingesting thousands of synthetic substances on a regular basis from the cradle to the grave, but then again it may not. Either way, the issue would not exist if these substances were not present in the first place. For instance, the conversion of methanol to formic acid mentioned above also happens in fizzy drinks. The beverage needs to be stationary for between 6 and 8 weeks at a temperature which exceeds 26.67°C (86 degrees F). Given that fizzy drinks are made to have a shelf life of up to six months, I think I'd be slightly concerned. If a person drinks more than three cans of a standard can of diet fizzy drink per day, they can experience a syndrome called metabolic [45] acidosis [46]. For ASP the syndrome will be caused by a build-up of formic acid in the general circulation. Studies and published papers funded by the manufacturers and protagonists behind ASP tend to suggest there is no risk. From this perspective the case is simple, the concentrations of aspartame consumed are tiny and the body can metabolise its break down products before they exert the kind of effects outlined above. ASP is not a toxin unless you ingest too much of it. On balance, the best way to avoid ASP is to remove it from your diet wherever and however you can. Now we can start to look into how ASP found its way into the Western diet. Clearly, the kind of criminal and self- serving activity detailed below is not unique to ASP. I would also argue that the events portrayed below are the norm and not the exception. Irrespective of context the story is the same it is merely the names which are different.

## Approving Aspartame

Once the sweet taste of aspartame had been discovered G.D. Searle began organising and then conducting field trials on ASP consumption, with a view to getting it approved as soon as possible. In pursuit of this objective, G.D Searle is alleged to have falsified or manipulated results. If that is the case then we are talking flat out fraud. Issues with the scientific case for approving ASP have been clear and present since before 1974. For example, in 1977 a document called the Bressler Report, (after its lead author Jerome Bressler who died on January 26th 2011) collated allegations of outright scientific fraud, irregularities inconsistencies and the deliberate falsification of results. As the last section in chapter five states and I reiterate here, more colloquially and outside of scientific circles we can be more forceful and call this behaviour *"pretending"*, *"cheating"* and *"lying"*, i.e. the basic foundations of any criminal behaviour. The Bressler report contains so many allegations that copies were sent to the offices of the District Attorney (DA) for the district of Chicago, a person called Samuel Skinner. The next step was going to be criminal charges all the way to the Grand Jury. All parties involved in the ASP fraud were to be tried and if found guilty prosecuted. Unfortunately for everyone who has ever been exposed to ASP in particular or uses sweeteners, the trial never happened. The Bressler Report was allegedly held under lock and key at the FDA for 30 years. If true, the obvious question is *"well, if you have nothing to hide why the secrecy?"* This quote from a now deceased Senator named Howard Metzenbaum [47] (Democrat Ohio) tells you all you need to know about how ASP got its approval. *"Searle, when making their presentation to the FDA, had willfully misrepresented the facts, and withheld some of the facts that they knew would possibly jeopardize the approval."* However at some time during the last months of 1976 or early 1977, Samuel Skinner withdrew from the case. According to the references, this happened after he had approved criminal action against G.D Searle. So, the obvious question is why? Well according to the *"literature"* he took on a senior position with a Chicago law firm called Sidley and Austin. Accordingly and despite the resignation of Skinner, the US Department of Justice (DOJ) pushed for the Grand Jury proceedings. This drive came from two sources, first, William Conlon (Skinner's temporary successor) and his permanent replacement Thomas Sullivan. Skinners new job was with Sidley and Austin who acted on behalf of G.D Searle. It is painfully predictable as to what happened next. The investigation into the dodgy science stalled [48] and a legal precedent called *"the statute of limitation [49]"* subsequently expired. Consequently, the entire investigation for criminal fraud against G.D Seale was unceremoniously dropped. Allegedly in December 1977, Thomas Sullivan ordered that the case be dropped for *"lack of evidence"*. At around this time, William Conlon also took employment with Sidley and Austin. A fully detailed and referenced report by Mr Metzenbaum alleges that the investigation into G. D. Searle was stymied and deliberately frozen so that time would run out and pass its statutory limit. At around the same time, an FDA employee a *"consumer product officer"* called Anthony Brunetti took a job within the food industry. He became a *"science adviser"* for an industry funded organisation called the *"soft drinks association"*. We are supposed to think that no conflict of interest exists with such developments, even though this particular move was cleared by the FDA itself. Really? Well, I beg to differ; Anthony Brunetti allegedly drafted the notices which led to the final approval of ASP in 1983. But there is no revolving door between big business, corporate funded science and regulatory approval is there? Oh no, and it gets better..........

All of this and other corporate shenanigans were occurring in the years before the election of Ronald *"raygun"* Reagan. For instance, Dr John Olney (whose discipline was neurology) of Washington / Iowa State University (now deceased [50]) had studied Multiple Sclerosis (with a view to curing it), mono-sodium glutamate and ASP since the 1970's. Research on ASP metabolism reveals that it causes or mimics the kind of symptoms and *"negative biological conditions"* outlined above. The research detailed by Dr Olney presents a litany of flaws with the research conducted by G D Searle. He also established that ASP can:

- Cause Brain tumours in laboratory animals
- Cause epileptic fits and eye damage in primates
- In higher concentrations, cause the formation of microscopic holes in the brains of laboratory rats
- And through the non-metabolism of phenylalanine led to an increase in the incidence of PKU

Needless to say, the usual suspects and those involved in getting ASP approved were fiercely critical and dismissive of such research. Now, I know who believe and I know who I stand with on such matters. Equally, I know why too! On this occasion, I stand with a world renowned and respected neuroscientist who has a stack of peer reviewed papers and equivalent publishing credits. I do not stand with those who have profited from the approval of ASP in particular and artificial sweeteners in general. Over the years 1975-80, the FDA itself was in broad agreement that ASP should not be in the food chain *"because it hasn't been demonstrated to be safe"*. A person called Alexander Schmidt who was an FDA commissioner ordered a re-assessment of 11 tests conducted by scientists employed by G.D. Searle. In 1976 he testified to the US Senate to the effect that ASP was unsafe and that the science supporting its safety credentials was unsound. In October 1980 the FDA's own public board of inquiry came to the same conclusion [51]. ASP should not by official approval have been allowed to enter the human food chain. The then chairman (Jere Goyan) of the FDA was to recommend further independent investigation and study of ASP. Around this time the FDA compelled G. D. Searle to desist from marketing ASP until such investigations were complete. Clearly, the wind was blowing against the current level of approval for ASP. However, the election of Ronald *"raygun"* Reagan to the mansion on the hill in November 1980 ensured that further evaluation of ASP never happened.

Aspartame and the *"Raygun"* Years

On January 21st 1981, Ronald Reagan was inaugurated as the 40th president of the United States. On the same date the former US secretary of defence, Donald *"rummy"* Rumsfeld suspended the authority of the commissioner of the FDA, Jere Goyan [52] who served under Jimmy Carter, the previous US president. At the time Donald Rumsfeld was CEO of G.D Searle but was also working as a key player in Ronald Reagan's transition [53] team. Clearly, there are no revolving door politics or conflicts of interest to consider here so the transparency continues. In February 1981 Arthur Hull Hayes [54] replaced Jere Goyan, as chair of the FDA; it appears, on the direct instruction of Donald Rumsfeld. It was Mr Hayes who went on to approve ASP, flying straight in the face of the FDA *"board of Inquiry"* position at the time that *"ASP is not safe, causes brain tumours and the position for approval is hereby revoked"*. As soon as ASP approval was granted, Mr Hayes went to work for a PR firm called Burston-Marsteller, being paid a thousand USD per day. Nice work if you can get it, and you don't have a conscience I guess. Mr Hayes is now deceased but had no experience of the science of food additives or their metabolism. Clearly, a perfectly sensible choice for chief decision maker inside the FDA! A pivotal reason for the replacement was to facilitate the approval of ASP. According to a blog in natural news [55] Jere Goyan was set to sign an FDA petition which would have revoked the approval for aspartame. Still, this wasn't enough because the FDA (again according to the literature) voted 3:2 against approving ASP. Arthur Hayes added a 6th and sympathetic member to the FDA approval board making the vote a tie. Then, (so the story goes) Arthur Hayes himself voted in favour of aspartame approval. I don't have much tuck with unfounded conspiracy theory. I also prefer to back up my assertions with some sort of evidence; otherwise, I am as bad as the Hayes and Rumsfeld's of this world. However, it would not surprise me at all if these kinds of maneuvers had occurred as stated above, with no grey areas and with no equivocations. The entire ASP story is riddled with corruption and conflicts of interest. These people and the construct they are part of have inflicted crystal clear and criminally unforgivable suffering on the peoples of the world. These mandarins of global power have directly contributed to the mass extinction levels of environmental destruction that is now unfolding before us. That is if you open your eyes to what is being done, has been done and about to happen toward, during and after 2020. Such people would think nothing of approving a potentially toxic synthetic compound, especially if they are to gain financially and politically. They see such approval as a means to an end, if they don't why, *"do they keep doing it (approving) for countless substances, lying about it, projecting outward about it and why do they keep doing very well out of it thank you very much?"*. If you needed any more convincing of how done up like a tin of sardines, such people have things, the patent on ASP was owned (via a subsidiary called the NutraSweet Company) by none other than G.D. Searle itself. Throughout the 1980's the NutraSweet company exclusively marketed ASP, after all this is what patents are for. The brand NutraSweet made hundreds of millions of dollars every year for about a decade on the back of the approval process. Hmmm, well I wonder? Could it be that the profit motive and some dodgy political maneuverings by some of the most loathsome people on the planet superseded sound and objective science as well as public health? I think so and in the strongest possible terms J'accuse the lot of them! If I'm wrong and there is nothing in all of this, I expect a summons for libel to be in the Vidda inbox by the end of 2017.

In July 1981 an FDA board of inquiry was set up to assess the safety of ASP once and for all. The board was populated by the best scientists in the agencies employ. At this time ASP was approved for sale and marketing only in dry foods. In the teeth of the above machinations the board was looking to present evidence that the approval of ASP ought to be revoked because it is *"unsafe and may cause brain tumors"*. Clearly, the revocation never happened. After the election of Ronald Reagan, the move to revoke was stymied by Mr Hayes, probably with the direct approval if not the explicit instruction of Mr Rumsfeld. By November 1983 aspartame was approved for use in soft and fizzy drinks. At which point both the Pepsi Cola and Coca Cola companies began using ASP in their products. Arthur Hayes was a professor and defence contract researcher and Donald Rumsfeld was a former secretary of defence. Wow! Stop, look, listen, can you smell the kippers? I can. The previous chairman of the FDA (Jere Goyan) was formally trained in pharmacology and was a passionate believer in patient rights. Professional attributes that neither Rumsfeld possesses nor Hayes possessed. Yes, for these people I do speak ill of the dead, why? They deserve it. By the end of 1983, Arthur Hayes was mired in scandal and resigned from the FDA. It was at this point that he took the PR job as a senior medical advisor with Burston-Marsteller. Not a bad position for a person with no moral or ethical code, understanding of nutrition, food science, biochemistry or pharmacology. During this period ASP was rebranded as NutraSweet and Canderel. A corporate solicitor called Robert Shapiro [56] came up with the brand name NutraSweet for ASP, the same Robert Shapiro who was CEO of

Monsanto from 1995 to the year 2000. The Monsanto company website publicly states [57] that they have not sold aspartame since the turn of the century. Mr Shapiro is also connected to that most criminal of organisations, *"The Bilderberg Group"* [58]. Over the 15 years from 1985 to the year 2000 the brand "NutraSweet" was owned by Monsanto. And it just goes on and on ad infinitum. Still, consumer choice has been upheld and money has been made, hasn't it? Hmmm, how pungent do those kippers smell now?

In the 1980's Donald Rumsfeld was Ronald Reagan's special envoy to the Middle East. Amongst his many nefarious roles was to legitimise relationships with Saddam Hussein. It was after this stint in global geopolitics that he returned to the top of G D Searle. In the middle [59] of 1985, the company was swallowed up (sorry purchased legitimately) by Monsanto for the tidy sum of 2.7 Billion dollars. As a result of the sale, Donald Rumsfeld received a bonus of 12 million dollars in the form of higher value stock options. It gets better, whilst he was the big cheese at G.D Searle Rumsfeld was awarded "outstanding [60] CEO of the year" in 1980 by the wall street transcript and another business orientated publication called financial world in 1981, such are the rewards for maximising profits. As an anti-war activist, I have learned how absolutely disgraceful and criminally psychopathic Donald Rumsfeld truly is. Sadly he is not alone and the mentality of the global elite he belongs to, permeates through every facet of our lives and ASP is but one consequence. Once you begin to look at how these people operate words simply are not enough. The debasement of people, planet and the environment is systemically criminal. Such benthic dwelling, detrivorous creatures should be sent to the ICC in The Hague where they can **ALL** tell us **ALL** about it in chains, in a prison uniform, in the dock. But, we do not live in such a world, instead, these people are allowed to profit from their crimes. The last time I saw Donald Rumsfeld was on the UK TV programme channel four news. He was deflecting questions about his past (these people always do) and talking about his latest venture, a war game app [61]. I guess if the cap fits, you have to carry on regardless of your glorification and acceptance of killing and destruction as the foundation of human nature. Thankfully most of humanity disagrees. And speaking personally by the time you read this book, I hope this particular verminous piece of human detritus will be where he belongs, dead in the ground or combusted in a crematorium. Either way, I don't care.

## Concluding Points

So, there we have it, the three questions at the end of paragraph one answered.

- ASP is a synthetic artificial sweetener discovered by accident
- It was approved as overviewed above
- Speaking personally, I would avoid it and all artificial sweeteners, should I/we/you be concerned? Well, do I/we/you trust the people involved in the approval process? There is your answer

ASP has been present in the human food chain since 1974 and the controversy surrounding it has not by one iota been settled if anything it has intensified. For example, papers published in 2011 hypothesise a direct correlation between ingesting ASP and liver and lung cancer in male mice. Research published in 2012 suggests links between ASP and blood cancers [62] (leukaemia, Non-Hodgkin lymphoma and multiple myeloma) in male laboratory animals. Despite the 2015 Pepsi Cola announcement and continual decreases in sales of fizzy drinks, ASP is still one of the most consumed food additives in the world. For example, the EU market [63] value for ASP in 2014 was just shy of £300 million. Although this figure looks set to drop to £210 million by the end of 2017, we are not talking about pennies in a piggy bank. This is big cash and it would be naïve to think that either ASP or the system which created it, developed, marketed it and continues to lie about it, is going away any time soon. A significant portion of the market value is fuelled by children and young people. ASP represents a confluence of bad science, insipid, biased and criminal regulatory practice, nepotism, corruption, nefarious financial dealings as well as shockingly self-serving political decision making. None of which surprises this writer!

We can safely conclude that from a purely scientific perspective that ASP is not the bogey man it has been made out to be. Conversely, it cannot by any means be considered safe for human consumption. In addition, the regulatory process itself clearly leaves huge space for improvement. As chapter three makes abundantly clear such improvement is not on the cards for the foreseeable future. For individuals, the only way to avoid ASP is to follow the advice presented in chapter three. Adopt a food orientated precautionary approach to these and other substances where ever you can. Whether the risks are real or not simply falls by the wayside if you are avoiding the substance(s) in question.

# Chapter Seven: Artificial Sweeteners

In a few years the year 2020 will be upon us. From climate considerations and the other factors mentioned at the start of chapter two, this period of time has always been something of a crunch point. As a species, especially in the western world, we have some serious decisions to make concerning our future on this Earth. Seriously, it really is "make our mind up time". And whatever happens, in the future, there will be no going back to how things were, the universe just does not work like that. We are now presented with an uncomfortable food reality that distils through every aspect of our lives. The insidiousness of this distillation displays itself as one bright shining consequence of how the food aspects of the modern world are now organised. Practically all of the food that most of us eat on a daily basis contains thousands of artificial substances. Many of which are novel or synthetic copies of naturally occurring nutrients. Most have been deemed safe for human consumption with no real assessment of their safety. Most have been added in secret, well away from the public domain. Certainly, most are added with no real scrutiny or awareness of their existence on the part of those who are ingesting them, i.e. you, I and most people on the planet. The processed food that most of us eat, most of the time, is not fit for purpose. This intensively made food is filled with substances that in some cases would not exist at all, were it not for the existence of the industry itself. Most have no business being in the food we eat. If the world were a different and better place, the synthetic substances (and plenty more besides), mentioned in this book would not be in our food, or anywhere else, period. The GRAS list (see chapter five) and classification by E number (see chapter five) indicate in crystal clear clarity that notions of safety are framed in terms which benefit the industry. The only factor that seems to matter is the quality of the science and how much of a given substance can be used without eliciting obvious harm. Humanity is now in a deplorable and criminal situation where thousands of substances are consumed simultaneously in tiny amounts by billions of people. If that reality does not represent a damning indictment of *"how things are done,* then I can be forgiven for asking *"what does?"* The industry has always lobbied and lobbied dirty against the existence and enforcement of the types of laws mentioned in chapter five. As the ongoing furore (well open political warfare) concerning the labelling of GM foods demonstrates, not very much has changed. And when change is foisted upon the food manufacturing industry it makes them for four basic reasons. Either new evidence, the availability of cheaper alternatives, hard campaigning or a combination of all three compels the industry to make some change or other. For instance, *"the Food Conspiracy"* book outlines how hydrogenated (saturated) fats and Trans-Fats have been replaced with slightly less damaging alternatives. Clearly, the factory scale bake-houses are not so keen to discuss why the fats are present in the first place. The same attitude permeates through the questions concerning artificial sweeteners in general. There are many dozens if not hundreds of substances that fall under the heading artificial sweetener. Aspartame discussed in chapter six is but one example. This chapter will highlight several more.

## High Fructose Corn Syrup (HFCS) and Sugar

One text book example of a substance that really ought not to be in the diet is high fructose corn syrup (HFCS [1]). It was developed in the late 1950's and since then its production around the world has sky rocketed. Outside of the circles populated by apologists for the industry HFCS is now recognised as one foundation of the global obesity epidemic. Despite the spin and distraction concerning this particular substance, the real reason HFCS is so popular with the processed food industry is that it is cheaper to make than sucrose. From the outset and until recently HFCS was promoted as a healthier alternative to sugar (sucrose). Fructose [2] ($C_6H_{12}O_6$) itself is another mono-saccharide carbohydrate which if eaten as part of a balanced diet is not particularly problematic. Fructose has the same formula as glucose but the atoms which make up the molecule are arranged differently. Glucose and fructose are isomers [3] of each other. The isomerism has various implications for both the sweetness and metabolism of each substance. Glucose is easier to metabolise than fructose, which is one reason why aerobic respiration prefers to use glucose as its primary source of energy. A third isomer of glucose is a substance called galactose. Fructose is found naturally in honey, sweet fruits and is a crucially important naturally occurring and sweet tasting molecule. However, HFCS is made from corn starch. The starch has been processed so that glucose derived from the starch is converted to fructose. The conversion happens due to the action of an enzyme [4] called glucose isomerase. The enzyme itself is not found in nature. It was developed in 1957 to specifically convert corn glucose to fructose. One cannot lay the blame for the global obesity epidemic at the doors of one substance, but HFCS is known to induce a syndrome called lipogenesis [5] in the liver. The quantities of fructose in HFCS cause the liver to overproduce fat, which does not form part of the job description of this crucially important organ. Lipogenesis causes a syndrome called non-alcoholic fatty liver disease (NALFD [6]) which is one of the most common diseases in the western world. It is also one of the most avoidable. Chapter three indicates the only true way to avoid ingesting HFCS, is to stop making it. As an individual, the best you can do is, avoid any food that contains it. Another factor concerning HFCS is biotechnology and genetic engineering as applied to food crops. In the United States HFCS is highly likely to be derived from genetically engineered corn. Needless to say, the biotechnology industry and associations which represent corn growers will tell you that GM corn is completely [7] safe. According to this agency, GM crops present no hazard to our health and will not damage the environment or cause any genetic pollution at all. Unsurprisingly, the reader should be aware that HFCS is on the GRAS list. HFCS is not a single molecule; there are several forms depending on the percentage of fructose each form contains. This partly explains why it has no designated e number. The industry is not required to label its products as containing HFCS even though it is present wherever an extra oomph of sweetness is needed. At an absolute minimum, a mandatory labelling regime for any food which contains HFCS is required. It is the absolute least that the industry could do. Yet, with reference to GMO's, I am not holding my breath in this area. One only has to look at aspartame (see chapter six) to understand that the movers and shakers in the food industry and its political backers simply cannot be trusted. Given the secrecy and prevalence of these molecules in the human food chain, people ought to be concerned. On a related point and one which underlines the label wash discussed in chapter two, in 2010 the industry proposed a name change for HFCS to corn sugar. In September 2017 there is no sign that HFCS will be banned or its production regulated. Several hundred thousand tonnes of HFCS are produced every year, most of it from the United States. Similarly, production in the EU looks set to triple in 2018. The syrup is used in fizzy drinks, sweets, cereal and dairy products. It is employed across the processed food industry to such an extent, that it is easier to say where it isn't used.

Table sugar or sucrose is a refined sugar. Each sugar molecule is made up of a molecule of glucose and one of fructose which are chemically bonded to each other. Before the body can use them they need to be broken down into their constituent molecules. Sucrose is also the base chemical for icing and caster sugar. The global consumption statistics [8] for refined sugar or sucrose are truly mind boggling. In the early 1960's the amount of sugar ingested by human beings was somewhere in the region of 60 million tonnes a year, by the turn of the 21st-century the figure was approaching 160 million tonnes. In 2017 the annual consumption of sugar is somewhere near 175 million tonnes. By far the biggest consumer of sugar and sugar products is the western world, with the US and UK being the two biggest single markets. The UK still eats more chocolate and confectionery products than any other European country. Very roughly about a quarter of the European market share is tied up with the UK. About 75% of all the sugar eaten in the UK is already in the processed food we eat. Avoiding excessive amounts of sugar is often problematic for a given population or individual. For the biochemical reasons which are outlined below, human beings like all animals including insects are attracted to sweet tasting foods. Animals interpret sweet tasting foods as a source of energy. The manufacturers are highly adept at distracting us from what is in the processed food they make, and sugar is no exception. The manufacturers are allowed to list the sugars separately and do not have to say that a particular compound is a sugar. The objective is to make the sugar content appear less than it is and they do not have to clearly state how much sugar a particular food contains. One tried and tested trick is to list sugars as carbohydrates and group both sets of molecules together. So for a given sugar containing product it is entirely possible to see X grams of carbohydrate per 100g of product. So, it is impossible to establish how much sugar a given product contains. Even when the sugar carbohydrate split is clearly stated the product is likely to contain glucose-fructose syrup plus sugar. The sugar content is often close to or above 50% of the carbohydrate total. Many high sugar processed foods are fortified (see chapter one) to make them appear more *"healthy"* than they are. Perhaps this is one reason why in 2004 Denmark [9] banned fortified foods. I'm sure there are other motivating forces behind such bans, but I am certainly not with the New York Times when it reports fortification [10] is a great idea. Nutrification (see chapters one and four) is a poor substitute for **NOT** processing perfectly natural wholesome, nutrient laden food in the first place. If food were not processed to the extent that it is, then fortification would not be necessary, another point missing from much of the discourse on this subject. Refined sugar is ubiquitous in the Western diet. Along with the obesity and diabetes epidemic, the presence of refined sugar in sweets and snacks has created a dental time bomb of equivalent, avoidable and epidemic proportions. Combine, sugars which are metabolised into acids by the action of bacteria in the mouth and reduced access to dental care with a lack of education and the teeth rot and dissolve, bingo! Aside from these considerations, sugar is big business, which means that sugar production is bad for the environment. All across the world sugar beet and sugar cane plantations represent a quintessential definition of the term *"environmental crime"*. From the destruction of rainforest to the extermination of the barrier reef, sugar is not good news. From water pollution and the destabilisation of the nitrogen [11] and phosphorous [12] cycles, the impact of sugar gets progressively worse. Here in the UK sugar beet production, distribution and marketing is controlled by a giant corporate entity called British Sugar. This operation is a wholly owned subsidiary of an even bigger conglomerate called *"Associated British Foods"*, who are mentioned in the Food Conspiracy book. British sugar has an annual turnover measured in hundreds of millions of pounds. They control about 60% of the entire UK sugar market and the UK's entire sugar beet quota. Most of this sugar is refined by Tate and Lyle who operate the only sugar refinery in the UK, located on the River Thames in East London; well they did until very recently. The refinery was sold to an American concern in 2010 [13]. The sale increased the value of Tate and Lyle shares from 10.4 to 460.1p, nice work if you can get it I guess! The refinery has the capacity to process over a million tonnes of sugar cane every year. OK, we have established that refined sugar is *"bad"* and HFCS is even worse. So all things considered perhaps artificial sweeteners are a better option? Well, let's see, shall we?

## Artificial Sweeteners and the Sugar Alcohols

From the outset, artificial sweeteners and the sugar alcohols (see below) have been promoted as a tried and tested method of cutting the calories without compromising on sweetness. The sweeteners are loosely defined as any substance used to sweeten a food instead of sugar (sucrose). Many thousands of compounds are classified as artificial sweeteners. None of these compounds exist in the natural world, they have all been produced in laboratories and most were discovered by accident. As far as our metabolism and the environment are concerned they are completely novel compounds. This reality has profound implications (see below) for the populations of microbes which call the human alimentary canal home. The manufacturers hold that artificial sweeteners are compounds which give an intensely sweet taste but do not add any calorific value to the diet. Plus, because they are so many times sweeter than sugar much less needs to be added to the food in question. By definition, artificial sweeteners cannot be considered food because they contain no nutrients and very few if any calories. They are often referred to as Non-Nutritive Sweeteners (NNS's). As far as we know most of them are not affected by digestive processes. They exist for one purpose and that is to act as a sugar substitute. All of this makes them a theoretical dead cert in the weight loss and diet stakes. They contain no carbohydrates and do not break down into glucose. This means they appear to be an attractive sugar substitute, especially if you are diabetic. Their sugar-free properties mean they can be found in sugar-free chewing gums and have been touted as a mechanism to improve dental health. In the US sweeteners are regulated by the FDA and reside in the GRAS list. In Europe regulation is through the EU where they have designated e numbers. These compounds can be hundreds of times sweeter than ordinary sugar. Some of the next generations of sweeteners are many thousands of times sweeter than sucrose. These latter substances have not been discovered by accident. Their inception, if it happens, will be deliberate and will fly in the face of the kind of research presented below. The NNS's are so intensely sweet that they need to be diluted with other substances, which the industry calls fillers. The fillers are needed so that the sweet taste does not overpower the sweet taste receptors on the human tongue. At this point, it is fair to present one spurious position the industry takes on artificial sweeteners. The manufacturers present their sweeteners as being calorie free. The use of fillers means that this is not the case. Dextrose [14] (which is a different form of glucose [15]) and maltodextrin [16] both work by bulking out a given quantity of sweetener. To really confuse matters dextrose and glucose are isomers [17] of each other, but dextrose is not an isomer of the other forms of glucose mentioned above. Dextrin (E 1400) and maltodextrin [18] are both used as food additives across the industry. Both of these compounds fall under the heading modified starch as discussed in chapter two. They are formed when starch is converted to sugar by means of hydrolysis reactions. These reactions break some of the glycosidic bonds which hold carbohydrates together. Starch molecules are broken down into simpler carbohydrate molecules. The fillers contain up to about a quarter of the calorific value of ordinary table sugar. If the sweetener you use contains such substances, then it cannot by definition be considered calorie free.

The NNS's only exist because the processed food industry has responded to our apparent demand for them. If this narrative is to be believed, people have wanted and then demanded low calorie but sweet foods. So, the food industry has responded by creating a whole plethora of NNS's. As the story behind aspartame demonstrates this is at best a false picture of how the NNS's came into existence. We the people have supposedly asked the industry to develop substances which satisfy our sweet tooth without running the risk of putting on the pounds, developing obesity or its bedfellow diabetes. This is just not the case. They were all discovered by accident in laboratories, patented and were then foisted upon the population as an alternative to sugar. If the reader is looking for one of the many bright shining lies which exemplify the operations of the processed food industry, then artificial sweeteners would be a good choice. As for notions of dealing with or preventing obesity, it is now becoming clear (see below) that the NNS's may well be contributing to and prolonging it, instead of helping to curtail it. Aside from the other points discussed below two additional factors (amongst the others) stood out:

- For a given quantity of sweetener, children carry about double the concentration in the blood stream than adults.
- The sweeteners find their way into breast milk [19] and so weaning mothers will be passing them and/or any metabolites on to their infants.

Children and infants are less able to remove sweeteners via the kidneys than adults can, so they will remain in the child's body for a longer time. As stated above the NNS's are wholly novel and synthetic. So we have no real base line to refer to concerning any impact they may have on the growth, development and taste preferences of a given child. However, given that it is well known that children generally like sweet foods more than adults do, they could be particularly vulnerable to any long term health impacts, should they present themselves.

Human beings have much in common with the other organisms which are alive on planet Earth. We breathe the same air, we have the same basic genetic code and we all respond to taste. We along with animals from insects to fish, other mammals and birds have a natural sweet tooth. We have evolved such that a sweet taste on the tongue is directly correlated with a source of energy (see below). It is this reality which forms the basis of a *"sweet tooth"*. People of all cultures, faiths, creeds and religions have been using *"natural sweeteners"* for thousands of years. However, the refined table sugars and highly processed substances, HFCS, sorbitol [20] (E 420 [21]) sucralose [22] (E 955), aspartame and plenty more besides, are a direct result of large scale food production. Aspartame is one example of the chemical difference between natural and artificial sweeteners; the other NNS's represent the other instances. The distinction between a natural and artificial sweetener is so clear that the two are entirely separate and mutually exclusive propositions. To suggest otherwise is to impart that chalk and cheese or hummus and guacamole are identical when clearly they are not. In the EU, 21 artificial sweeteners are approved for human consumption. They range from E 420 to E 969 [23], including several sugar alcohols [24]. The most abundant sugar alcohols in the Western diet are:

- Erythritol [25] (E 968)
- Glycerol (E 422 [26])
- Isomalt [27] (E 953 [28])
- Lactitol [29] (E 966 [30])
- Mannitol [31] (E 421) [32]
- Sorbitol,
- Xylitol [33] (E 967 [34])
- Hydrogenated starch hydrolysates (HSH)

The sugar alcohols are sweet tasting carbohydrates found naturally in fruits and berries. They are also known as hydrogenated carbohydrates. Various chemical processes are employed to extract a purified form of the sugar alcohol in question. For instance, xylitol is extracted from xylan [35] which is produced when wood pulp is used to make cellulose (see chapter one). Xylan is another long chain carbohydrate molecule and a key component of the plant cell wall. Xylitol is also found in fruits and berries and does have well established medicinal uses. For example, it is extracted from birch wood and is used to treat mild ear infections in children. As with the other artificial sweeteners Xylitol is presented as an alternative to refined sugar. It is also known to inhibit the growth of bacteria on the teeth and gums, so, it is used in dental treatment [36]. Glycerol is produced from propene or from the fermentation of sugars. Propene is derived from the breakdown of much larger compounds in crude oil. It is likely that the glycerol found in food is likely to be sourced from the petrochemical industry. Or it may well come from the sugars derived from genetically engineered corn crops. Or, equally likely, both! Genetically Modified (GM) corn and petrochemicals are the two primary sources of all the sugar alcohols in the human food chain. That seems reason enough to avoid them where ever possible. As compounds, the sugar alcohols are classified as polyols. These are substances which contain two or more alcohols. Aside from food processing, they have application in cosmetics, medicine and pharmaceuticals. You may see a family of chemicals which are related to sugar alcohols and artificial sweeteners. The Hydrogenated Starch Hydrolysates [37] (HSH) molecules are essentially various hybrids of the sugar alcohols or other alcohols. They are also used as bulking agents and/or to add texture and thickness to a given food. All of these substances are considered safe at the levels present in the western diet, all have e numbers and all have been petitioned by the industry as being suitable for the GRAS list (see chapter five). The sugar alcohols and HSH compounds are used as sweeteners and sugar substitutes; they are anywhere from about half to three-quarters as sweet as refined table sugar. They have little (if any) calorific or nutritional value and are used in conjunction with much sweeter artificial sweeteners, i.e. they are also used as fillers. The human digestive system struggles to break down the sugar alcohols. For instance, at present, the bacteria in our mouths cannot touch them. They remain unchanged and so sugar-free chewing gum manufacturers employ them as a substitute for sugar (sucrose). However, with the exception of erythritol which remains unchanged, if ingested the bacteria in the colon can and do ferment the sugar alcohols. The fermentation has been known to cause flatulence, bloating and abdominal pain. Some of the sugar alcohols can stimulate diarrhoea and intensify (but not cause) existing syndromes including Irritable Bowel Syndrome (IBS). For people who suffer from these conditions, the diet has to be monitored. The sugar alcohols used in food manufacturing are derived from industrial processes and so cannot be considered as natural ingredients. They are also used as gels, emulsifiers, stabilisers and thickeners. The different utility of these compounds explains the wide range of e numbers. An industry website called polyols EU gives an overview of the industrial uses and how the food manufacturers view the application of the polyol compounds. As usual the *"why are they added to the food we eat?"* question, is missing from the industry narrative.

For several decades artificial sweeteners have been presented as a *"healthy"* substitute for *"unhealthy"* sugar (sucrose). This explains why they are found mainly in diet and reduced calorie foods. Perhaps the most familiar artificial sweeteners are aspartame, neotame, saccharin and sucralose. Up until very recently, it was assumed that as a class of compounds they are chemically inert. The best of both worlds could present itself. A person could get the sensation of sweetness, without eating nasty bad refined sugar, lose weight and still eat a bit of what they fancy without putting on the pounds or kilos. A person can satisfy their sweet tooth without the negative health impacts of refined sugar or HFCS. However, it is now emerging that the NNS's are not as chemically inert as was previously assumed. Now, why am I not surprised? So what is happening to the sweeteners in the bodies of people who ingest them? Well, the real truth is that we do not know the precise metabolic pathways of these compounds. That being the case, science has established some broad strokes which will in time I believe completely change how people view them. A few of these broad strokes are presented below.

## Artificial Sweeteners Diet and Microbes

It is becoming apparent that sweeteners can have a direct impact on the metabolic and homeostatic balance of human beings and other animals. Artificial sweeteners are absolutely novel, they are wholly synthetic compounds. The latest 2017 research indicates that the communities of microbes inside us have the ability to respond to the presence of NNS's. This should not surprise anybody. Microbes can and do respond to the presence of new substances in their environment. Aside from any other points, microbes are always looking for new sources of chemical energy to drive their metabolism. If they are receiving a daily dose of novel chemicals in the form of artificial sweeteners it stands to reason that they will over time respond biochemically. Whether the response is beneficial or dangerous to us will not be of the slightest concern to the microbes in question. If they can grasp an opportunity to outperform their neighbours they will take it and use it to their advantage. The section on fruit juice in chapter four highlights the adaptability of microbes to changing circumstances. In addition to these potential biological impacts, it now appears that artificial sweeteners can induce the very set of symptoms [38] they are supposed to prevent. At no point should the reader go away from this chapter thinking that using artificial sweeteners is definitely going to cause harm or damage. However, the evidence has been presented for several decades [39] and the research continues at apace. The Nature Publishing Group and The Lancet are not bastions of political activity and campaigning are they? I am but they are not. So, if science journals with highbrow reputations concerning the assertions they make are expressing concern about an issue it would be good practice to hear what the research has to say for itself. The clear and present conflicts of interest between the industry position and its bottom line are just as apparent as they have always been. Clearly, things are swirly and murky in the world of artificial sweeteners and in recent years things have gotten even swampier.

It is clear that sweeteners [40] could be intensifying the wholly preventable global obesity and diabetes epidemic. In 2014 it became clear through work published in the science journal nature (and others) that sweeteners could be causing microbes in our guts to provoke glucose intolerance in susceptible individuals. The intolerance happens when the blood glucose level is high enough for a long enough time such that the body cannot cope with it. Glucose intolerance lays the foundation for obesity and type-2 diabetes. Based on such findings there are calls a plenty to re-assess the status of the artificial sweeteners highlighted in this chapter. Nobody in the scientific establishment saw it coming because it *"never occurred"* to anyone to look at this particular metabolic pathway. This mantra presents itself every time the industry is caught out when it is shown that a substance it has designated as safe, turns out not to be so. Glucose intolerance means that an affected individual cannot metabolise glucose and so this simplest of carbohydrates begins to build up in the blood stream. The syndrome is called hyperglycemia and is generally seen as a stepping stone to full blown type 2 diabetes. Just to confuse matters, (I mean it would be rude not to), it is now clear that artificial sweeteners can trigger a spike in insulin production, whose action provokes the formation of glycogen (glycogenesis [41]). It could be that the NNS's could be upsetting the mechanisms which enable us to regulate our appetite and feeding habits.

The Medicine on your plate series of books discusses diabetes in some detail. Monosaccharides are made up of one carbohydrate molecule, with glucose and fructose being the most familiar. Glucose is the primary energy source which drives our metabolism and that of most organisms on the Earth. The body uses it directly as soon as digestion makes it available. Any excess is converted to a long chain carbohydrate molecule called glycogen. Glycogen is stored in the liver until it is needed. When the blood sugar level drops below a certain concentration (which varies from person to person), the glycogen is broken down via the action of a hormone called glucagon. This action releases glucose back into the bloodstream. At its absolute simplest glucagon works in the opposite way to insulin. With hyperglycemia induced by glucose intolerance, the stored glucose is converted straight to fat bypassing the formation of glycogen (glycogenesis). On top of that, people with hyperglycemia often develop higher blood pressure, arterial and heart disease which can lead to stroke and/or heart attacks. It gets worse; the same research indicates that even when healthy individuals who have no history of glucose intolerance ingest saccharine and other artificial sweeteners, some do begin to express hyperglycemic symptoms. It must be stressed that equally compelling and rigorous research suggests that NNS's when consumed by healthy lean individuals elicit none of the negative symptoms mentioned in this chapter. Having highlighted this point the basic conclusion from this emerging corpus of research is equally valid. If you are already overweight, a person is likely to adopt a prescribed diet of one form or another. If that diet were to include substitutes for sugar and you were susceptible to glucose intolerance, you could well find yourself hit with a double whammy in the weight (mass) loss department. Nothing here is categorical, but the research is progressing. So, what is the research telling us about the metabolism of artificial sweeteners?

Microorganisms are not passive. They will respond to stimulus and chemical changes in their environment. It is this ability which makes them so adaptable. The NNS's are not usually absorbed into the blood stream but they do come into contact with the literally trillions of individual microbes in our intestines. The research in question suggests that the microbes are reacting to the presence of long term consumption of artificial sweeteners. The implication is that the biochemistry of these populations changes to accommodate the presence of novel chemicals in their habitat. The implied result is a proclivity for obesity and all the syndromes associated with it. The microbes will not be concerned with any such consequences. This research is based on the results of experiments carried out on laboratory rodents. I am not in any way suggesting that the same pathway definitely occurs in human beings. Similarly, none of this should suggest that the artificial sweeteners are unique in their ability (to potentially) upset the microbial balance of the human alimentary canal. Eating intensively produced foods has been shown to impact negatively on the metabolism, diversity and growth of bacteria in the human gut. That being made clear, I do believe in the precautionary principle and this would be enough for me to dispense with artificial sweeteners immediately.

The largest human trial that I am aware of carried out in this area falls under the banner of a project called the personal nutrition project, their website is listed below. It has been going on since 2014. The trial is still open to new participants, so please do feel free to have a go! The project seeks to establish to what extent (if at all) nutrition affects the community of microbes in the human alimentary canal. One aspect of the study found that even after just one week of ingesting the sweeteners available some participants did begin to develop glucose intolerance. The basic hypothesis concludes that in susceptible individuals their intestinal bacteria react to the sweeteners by secreting substances which provoke an inflammatory or allergic response which is similar to a *sugar overdose*. Ultimately, those affected lose the ability to properly metabolise glucose and express varying degrees of glucose intolerance. Given that the marketing and development of artificial sweeteners is pretty much unregulated, such conclusions ought to be raising eyebrows, whether you ingest artificial sweeteners or not. The basic reason people use NNS's is to lose weight, cut out the calories or just because a person does not like sugar. So, it should elicit further questions from the reader, if it came to pass that sweeteners stimulated appetite as well as glucose intolerance. A definite potential perfect negative storm if there ever was one! However, it is entirely likely that neither [42] could occur or that intolerance and appetite stimulation could manifest separately. The simple truth is that we just don't know either way, but we can say that such metabolic impacts could occur. We can say that researchers have established a mechanism through which sweeteners can affect the way the brain regulates taste, its interpretation and then a person's appetite. We just don't know exactly what the mechanism is, just that it is there. This particular body of research also looked at how the brain associates the sweetness and energy content of ingested foods. Again, the research was based on vivisection experiments. In this case, that favourite of initial research programmes, the humble Drosophila melanogaster, or the common fruit fly. [43] Given this research was carried out in 2016 it is very early days. The expression *"take this with a pinch of salt"* is a bit Diana Ross, in that it is supremely relevant. The research indicates that long term ingestion of a diet containing *"normal"* levels of sucralose, will lead to the flies consuming more sucralose than they did previously. The research concludes that the sensation of *"sweetness"* is firmly integrated with the brain's interpretation of energy content. Such that *"the sweeter"* an ingested food is, the greater the degree the brain will associate it with increased energy content. The research is suggesting that when the *"sweetness"* and *"energy"* relationship is skewed the brain resets itself and the body begins to crave more food. In this experiment, the fruit flies which had the enhanced sucralose diet consumed 30% more calories than those which were fed naturally sweet food sources.

If you think about it, this makes perfect sense. Glucose is the simplest carbohydrate and is the source of energy which drives the respiration of every aerobic organism on the Earth. That span of organisms covers the microbial world, the insect world, the mammalian world and every living organism in between. Most of the organisms which call the Earth home respire aerobically. So it is not unrealistic to suppose that the same kind of associations that exist in fruit flies will also exist (but will be infinitely more complex) in human beings. The assertion is that long term ingestion of artificial sweeteners tricks the brain into *"thinking"* that even natural sweet substances are sweeter than they are. The brain *"thinks"* these substances contain glucose and other simple sugars when they don't. Perhaps billions of people consume NNS compounds. Yet science is just beginning to really understand their metabolic impact and their role in appetite and feeding. This research suggests that an organism's brain will respond to artificial sweeteners by tricking the body into thinking it needs more energy than it really does and the urge to eat is intensified. All points considered, the availability of NNS's in the western diet seems to stimulate the urge to eat and the stimulus is not switched off. Clearly, such an eventuality would at the very least represent one foundation of the global obesity crisis. A system induced epidemic which blights the lives of hundreds of millions of people all over our world.

## Psychology, Hormones and Obesity

Another factor which is often ignored in helping obese people is the notion of eating addiction as opposed to food addiction per se. Unless there is a prescribed medical condition people who do over eat or are obese are not dependent on a single ingredient. What tends to happen is that people in this bracket may well remove sugar or HFCS from their diet, but will compensate by eating other foods. The kind of foods in question are the highly refined, energy dense, nutritionally deficient convenience or fast variety which are available everywhere across the western World, but in particular the US and UK. Here we are looking at the "pleasure-reward" [44] cycle and a loss in the ability to control or eliminate an activity which is doing harm to the person concerned. The references below presents the research which shows that *"food dependency"* elicits a more powerful response in susceptible individuals than cocaine and heroin addiction does. Further research [45] carried out in Australia in 2016 indicates that insects fed a diet rich in sucralose for five days became hyperactive and glucose intolerant as compared to control groups. Similar research carried out by the same team on rodents led to identical conclusions. This area of research is continually growing. The 2016 study concludes that the neural circuitry regulating *"pleasure-reward cycle"* is re-aligned. In this research ingesting sucralose switched on a pathway that normally operates when the organism is hungry and it doesn't switch off. The urge to eat becomes over riding and relentless. The Lancet or the nature publishing group are not known for making wild unfounded assertions and they certainly do not live in wild unfounded conspiracy theory land. Such organisations deal in *"objective science"* intertwined with *"robust and evidence based conclusions"*, so if the science is wrong or inaccurate or flawed in some way, it doesn't get published, certainly not by these and equivalent journals. Now, we cannot compare insects with rodents on a like for like basis any more than you can compare both sets of organism with human beings. What you can say is that if it occurs in one organism then there is no reason to suppose that it doesn't in another. After all, organisms use the same basic hormones and neurological signals to carry out their metabolic and life processes as well as to respond to the world around them. It is in the teeth of such findings that the food industry, various trade associations and the science they fund attempts to dispute the above conclusions or try to frame the health consequences as someone else's fault. They are seeking to deny and deflect their own culpability and responsibility. In my experience, such behaviour only presents itself when an organisation has something to hide. Once again, when the usual vested interests and bucket loads of cash come into the picture responsibility for consequences is deflected, projected and denied, no change there then. Conversely, emerging research suggests that an opposite strategy might be more useful in shedding the weight and maintaining a given dietary regime. Here it is important to stress the language, the terms *"early days"* or *"the results are confusing or conflicting"* are there for a reason. Bitter tasting foods and so by association any "bitter" dietary supplement may be more effective in curtailing undesirable eating habits.

The sensation of feeling hungry is in part caused by the action of a hormone called ghrelin.[46] As far as glucose and amino acids are concerned when they are in the stomach specialist receptors are activated. The activation triggers the release of ghrelin. In human beings, ghrelin encourages appetite and feeding. However, when bitter sensations are detected after about 30 minutes the urge to eat is decreased and the body has a tendency to keep digesting food in the stomach for much longer periods of time. The appetite is curtailed and we have the *"full-up"* sensation much quicker than we would normally. This is the conclusion [47] of recent research in this area. We now know that various receptors are distributed throughout the intestines. These specialist cells are believed to influence appetite and the activity of various digestive and other hormones. It is not outside the bounds of possibility that such activity could have game changing bearings on treating obesity. Having said that, surely a better bet is to deal with their causes and not focus exclusively on the consequences. Obesity is characterised by profound biochemical changes in the body. The metabolic balance of the body is skewed to such an extent that a new homeostatic balance is established. Fat cells become the norm and they proliferate and then they proliferate some more. The brain engages in profound and intense dopamine [48] signalling and the *"pleasure – reward"* cycle goes into overdrive. Here, when a person *"goes on a diet"* the body acts as if it is being deprived of food. The desire to eat intensifies and ultimately becomes irresistible. We have all done it; we have all eaten more than we should have done, especially if what we are eating is particularly tasty. Now imagine you have that urge all the time and there is lots of what you fancy right in front of you, every day and everywhere you go. Even if this stratospherically high metabolic hurdle is passed things don't get any easier. Once a person has shed the extra mass they have to eat significantly less and keep doing so more than most other people. Even then, the urge to over eat does not really dissipate. If this is really what is going on with the metabolism of obese people it is little wonder that it so difficult to treat and that relapses are so common. When the food desert and food bank statistics and availability of processed food is factored into such a relationship, it seems obvious that dealing with obesity in any *"Western"* population becomes an exercise in criminal dysfunction. It would seem that the best way to avoid obesity and its precursor conditions is to stop manufacturing so much of the food that is implicated in its cause. However, that objective requires the kind of solution alluded to in chapter three and I see no sign of that happening, not for the foreseeable future. Intertwined with this position would be establishing a real connection between people and food and where it comes from. Perhaps the food for life partnership (whose website is listed below) ought to be rolled out on a national scale. Sadly, such demonstrably successful initiatives have been totally gutted by cuts under the banner of austerity.[49] A paltry £1.25 million [50] grant from the big lottery fund is an insult. I'm sure the soil association (whose website is listed below) will make good use of it, but please, let's get real shall we?

The above discoveries have caused all sorts of problems for the food industry in general and for the makers of the NNS's in particular. We are not as yet at a stage where a causative link between ingesting artificial sweeteners by individuals who are susceptible to glucose intolerance and obesity can be established. I am also sure that the European Food Safety Authority (EFSA) and others will rigorously review the status of sweeteners. They will also do this diligently and methodically but I'm willing to bet they will look only at individual compounds in isolation from the rest of the diet. They will also be seeking to establish new acceptable limits of safety. They will also look at any next generation sweeteners in the same manner and will not consider that the substances themselves should not exist and are but one component of the collection of chemicals we call additives. In any case, I will not be holding my breath for the industry to make any future declaration concerning the negative health impacts of NNS's. There is simply too much money and vested interest at stake. The global market for artificial sweeteners is measured in hundreds of millions of dollars and so they like processed foods are not going away any time soon.

## Sucralose

We have all seen sucralose marketed in crystalline powdered form, in pretty little yellow packets [51] as a sweetener called Splenda. As the name suggests it is derived from sucrose. It was discovered in 1976 by food scientists in the employ of Tate and Lyle. Sucralose has been approved by regulatory authorities in 60 different countries. It is found in over 3000 individual products ranging from soft drinks to desserts and dairy products, meaning sucralose is everywhere. The molecule is about 600 times sweeter than sugar. Like most of the approved artificial sweeteners sucralose does not generally break down in the body. When ingested approximately 85% passes straight through the digestive system. The remainder is absorbed into the general circulation. Sucralose does not readily accumulate in the body. However, none of this means that sucralose is biologically inactive; a peer reviewed assessment [52] published in 2014 states that sucralose:

- Reduces the numbers and balance of bacteria in the human intestine.
- Can pass into the bloodstream.
- Can scar the internal surface of the intestine and damage or deplete the numbers of specialist cells there.
- Can act as mutagens on the cells of the human intestine.
- Can alter the levels of glucose and insulin in the bloodstream.
- Produces a whole range of unknown novel metabolites when the absorbed portion is broken down.
- Can interfere with the uptake and mode of action of medicinal drugs.
- If used in baking can decompose into compounds called

chloro-proponals,[53] which may be both carcinogenic and genotoxic

This particular body of research concludes that at the very least a thorough re-assessment of the safety of sucralose and any foods which contain it is urgently required. Based on that list I would be inclined to agree. I would like to think that any sensible person would take it upon themselves to investigate further, especially if they ingest sucralose regularly. Sucralose is also believed to increase the pH level (making it more alkaline) of the human alimentary canal. It is also believed to be absorbed by fat cells. Should those fat cells be metabolised (which if you are overweight they ought to be) the sucralose will also be released back into the bloodstream.

Sucralose is marketed as being safe for its intended use and in normal concentrations [54] even when consumed for long periods of time.[55] The official line is that when it is consumed on its own a person would have to ingest large amounts of sucralose to elicit any toxic effect. The quantities consumed on each occasion are indeed tiny. However, we do not consume these substances in isolation from each other, quite the opposite occurs. We consume additives and sweeteners, in tiny concentrations, in combination with thousands of other substances over periods of time measured in decades. We have no real idea how such substances will interact with each other. How can we know? No human population has ever regularly consumed so many different synthetic substances at any point throughout our history. This fact is ignored wholesale by every single regulatory authority on the planet. Food processing in its current form represents food poisoning on a global scale. On that basis alone j'accuse [56] and I do so in the strongest possible terms. Much of the science concerning the safety of sweeteners in particular and additives in general looks only at short term studies where large doses of single chemicals are administered to laboratory animals. Such scenarios are the complete opposite of what happens in the real world. If I was to submit a paper for review on this basis I would be wide open to accusations of scientific fraud (i.e. lies) and justifiably and rightly so. It should not surprise the reader to realise that the bodies responsible for protecting public health generally do not demand the necessary holistic scientific study. There is no pressure on them to consider other factors, so they don't, it truly is that simple. All of this can be made a moot if simplistic point by once again adopting your very own personal precautionary principle. If you don't want to run the risk of any adverse toxic effects, whether they are real or not, avoid artificial sweeteners.

Assertions of safety also tend to dismiss anecdotal or evidence based on testimony of harm from individuals as *"unscientific"* or alarmist. The very real concerns that a given population has over a given set of chemicals are dismissed by the scientific establishment. This condescending attitude from so many professional scientists really does annoy and upset this writer in equal measure. As the name suggests it is true that Sucralose is made from sucrose (sugar). Yet that is it, from a chemical perspective sucralose is as close to sugar as rock music is to kraftwerk. Sucrose is a di-saccharide with the formula $C_{12}H_{22}O_{11}$ made of two glucose molecules which are chemically bonded to each other. Sucralose is a chlorinated form of sucrose with the formula $C_{12}H_{19}Cl_3O_8$. Sucralose production is a hidden and closely guarded process. The conversion of sucrose to sucralose is a five step process protected by patent law, which converts sucrose into a molecule which is not found anywhere in nature.

The sucrose molecule contains several structures called hydroxyl (OH) groups. This structure is composed of one atom of hydrogen and one atom of oxygen which are chemically bonded to each other. To make sucralose three of these structures are removed and replaced with atoms of chlorine. The source of the chlorine atoms is phosgene gas [57] ($COCL_2$), the same substance that was used alongside mustard gas [58] during the First World War. This is not unusual because phosgene is used in the production of dyes, pesticides and various forms of plastic.

Treating sucralose with phosgene produces a compound called 1,6-dichloro-1,6-dideoxy-beta-D-fructofuranosyl-4-chloro-4-deoxy-alpha-D-galactopyranoside. A water soluble chlorinated hydrocarbon called sucralose. The presence of the chlorine atoms has drawn parallels with perhaps the most infamous chlorinated hydrocarbon of them all, the insecticide Dichloro-Di-phenyl-Trichloroethane (DDT [59]). Sucralose is not in the same league of toxicity as the organochlorine [60] pesticides. Some would say the two play entirely different sports and one always has to get the science right. However, just because a comparison may not be valid on a like for like basis, does not mean other issues [61] are invalid. For instance, it is becoming clear that chlorinated sweeteners will degrade on heating and release individual chlorine atoms into baked goods. The free chlorine atoms are then able to recombine with other atoms in the food forming the potentially toxic chloro-propanols mentioned above. So, on that basis alone, sucralose may not be as safe as the manufacturers and some scientists say it is.

Such realities are not supposed to bother us. Tate and Lyle who manufacture sucralose maintain that it is a chemically inert compound which passes through the body without being metabolised or broken down. However, there is no such thing as a completely stable compound, under the right conditions any substance will react with its surroundings. If we accept that 15% of ingested sucralose makes its way into the general circulation then it stands to reason that some of this quantity will undergo some form of chemical change, especially if a person is ingesting it regularly as one component of their diet. One substance that has been associated with sucralose storage and metabolism is a substance called 1,6 di-chloro-fructose. It is unclear, through a lack of testing whether this substance exhibits any toxic effect. At the time of writing, Sucralose metabolism has also been implicated in reducing the size and activity of the thymus gland [62] and the spleen.[63] It has also been suggested that elevated levels of sucralose can increase the size of the liver and result in stunted growth rates for both children and infants. Sucralose is approved for use as a sweetener and I'm sure the 110 plus studies submitted by Tate and Lyle facilitated the process. Needless to say, these studies concluded the safety of sucralose by one mechanism or another. The FDA approved sucralose in 1999, in 2004 the EU followed suit.

Sucralose is perhaps best known under the brand name Splenda a brand whose turnover is worth hundreds of millions of currency units to its manufacturer [64] Heartland Food Products. A study carried out in 2013 at Washington University found that sucralose alters the mechanism by which the body deals with sugar. This particular study involved 17 severely obese people with no history of diabetes and who have no history of regular sweetener use. The study found that in the human digestive system, sucralose is not inert. The research team was very quick to point out that *"more study"* is needed to determine whether or not long term use is dangerous to human health. Since 2013 the scientific community has kindly obliged in this endeavor. In 2017 plenty of research is available which at the very least begins to question the role of sweeteners in the human diet. As time passes the corpus of objective knowledge will increase! Simultaneously, corporate sponsored science will seek to impart that all is well and good. The 2013 Washington study concludes that the consumption of sucralose was *related to an enhanced blood insulin and glucose response"*. In this regime, the participants responded by releasing the appropriate amount of insulin, so that the body becomes neither hyperglycemic (too much glucose) or hypoglycemic (too little glucose). The body responded as it should to increases and decreases in blood sugar levels. However, if the long term presence of sucralose (and other sweeteners) in the diet promotes the release of insulin, the body may not respond to insulin as it should and that can lead to type-2 diabetes. It is not so much the sweetener that is provoking the enhanced response, but more the response from the brain when it interprets intense sensations of sweetness and how that upsets the sweetness energy relationship outlined above.

## Neotame

Chemically neotame [65] is similar to aspartame and is up to 13,000 times as sweet as ordinary sugar, yes you read that right! The chemical formula for Neotame [66] is $C_{20}H_{30}N_2O_5$ and it looks set to become the replacement for aspartame. Chemically there is not much to distinguish the two compounds. However, neotame is more stable and heat resistant and breaks down less readily than aspartame. For the industry, it is attractive because it has none of the PKU problems associated with its predecessor (see chapter six). It is also much more stable than aspartame. Likely, the industry will not be required to label any foods as containing it and it will probably turn up wherever heat resistant sweeteners are needed. The stability difference is due to the presence of a substance called 3, 3-dimethyl-butyl. This extra molecule prevents the breakup of neotame and stops the release of phenylalanine, the amino acid which causes PKU in susceptible people. In its pure form neotame is highly flammable and an irritant, it also has a variety of warnings concerning how it can be used and how it ought to be handled. Aside from the presence of the butyl molecule neotame and aspartame are essentially the same substance. However, because of the butyl group, neotame does not break down into methanol when ingested. Plus unlike aspartame, it can remain unchanged for months or even years in the cans which contain soft drinks. Which will extend their shelf and transportation life. This is another reason why neotame is attractive to the industry. The extra life will lead to lower costs and increased profits. Neotame has the number e 961 and is about 30 times as sweet as aspartame. Neotame is made by NutraSweet (who also make aspartame) and in a very real sense is marketed as a substitute for aspartame. The reader can clearly infer that no conflict of interest declaration is warranted. Demonstrating its loyalties, the US FDA has suggested that no labelling for the presence of neotame is needed. It was granted approval for use as a food additive in the EU in 2010.[67] Neotame is found in frozen desserts, some chewing gums, sweet baked foods, breakfast cereals and some spreads. It also has utility as a flavour enhancer and is one of those sweeteners to look out for. Neotame is on its way to a processed food near you and it will be there soon if it isn't already. However, do not expect this to be stated on the label. As neotame is so much sweeter than aspartame in theory less of it should be needed to instil a given degree of sweetness. This argument is used as justification for introducing it to the human food chain. In this context, because less of it is needed the potential for toxicity should be reduced. The industry is less keen impart that as a result of its intense sweetness neotame could well find utility across the food manufacturing industry. This should cause concern because neotame may well be more neurotoxic, excito-toxic and immuno-toxic than aspartame ever was. Just don't expect NutraSweet or any other agency which will gain from neotame to admit it.

The very real concerns surrounding artificial sweeteners in general also apply to neotame. The same substances that are present in aspartame also exist in neotame. The main substances in question are aspartic acid and phenylalanine. These two amino acids are believed to influence how leptin and insulin operate in the body. Both of these hormones regulate metabolism and are involved with how the body stores fat and whether or not we feel hungry. It is becoming clear that consumption of artificial sweeteners can raise insulin and leptin levels. Increased levels of both of these hormones are directly correlated with obesity and therefore all of its bedfellows. When the body is burdened by elevated leptin levels the hormonal signals to stop eating become disrupted, fat cells are less likely to break down and the sweet signalling pathways discussed elsewhere in this chapter become skewed. The resulting leptin resistance means that the body produces and stores more fat cells and cravings for sweet tastes become over whelming. Leptin intolerance is another mechanism by which the body becomes tricked into thinking it is hungry when it is not. Once again we are confronted by a wholly avoidable set of symptoms caused by obesity. The industry and proponents of artificial sweeteners will disregard these assertions and present data and experiments which impart that neotame is *"safe, well tolerated and not associated with any adverse health impacts"*, even when the experimental doses are *"15 times the projected daily consumption by high-level consumers"*. So that's that settled, I'll disregard the precautionary principle along with the notion that neotame and other equivalent substances should not exist and I'll start on the neotame. Sorted!

## Saccharine

Saccharine [68] is the oldest sugar substitute on the planet. It was discovered in 1879 and has a history of controversy which rivals that of aspartame. It is designated as E 954 [69] and is produced industrially from a precursor compound called toluene,[70] which at high concentrations is a potential carcinogen [71]. Toluene ($C_6H_5CH_3$ [72] or $C_7H_8$) is a widely used solvent which can and does have various toxic impacts on the human central nervous system. It should not surprise the reader to find that since the 1970's saccharin has been implicated in carcinogenesis [73] in male laboratory rats. The amounts necessary to induce cancer are relatively high; something the industry has seized upon to bolster its *"saccharin is ok"* position. However, as those scientists who spoke out in favour of a ban point out, it is children who are going to be most vulnerable to any saccharin induced cancer. They are still growing and are more likely to ingest the sweets and soft drinks which contain saccharin and the other approved sweeteners. So what does any self-respecting profit making enterprise do in response? It buys the law and it lobbies, that's what it does! The industry, in the form of a trade body called the Calorie Control Council, fought hard to get saccharin removed from any statute linking the sweetener with cancer. Such criminal self-interest ought to be seen in conjunction with the removal of statutes, exemplified by the Delaney clause (see chapter six). A US scientific body called the National Toxicology Programme has lobbied and voted such that in the US saccharin is listed as an *"anticipated human carcinogen"*. [74] Surprisingly, saccharine was banned in the US over the years 1981 until 2010. As for Europe, in 2013 The EFSA declared saccharin (and aspartame) as safe for human consumption and have even suggested that its consumption ought to be encouraged. Saccharin is found in sugar-free chewing gums and dental health products. Saccharin is an NNS and is used in over 100 countries. The industry position and that of many scientists is that because a person would need to eat impossibly huge amounts of foods containing saccharin that the ban is unnecessary. Again they deny or miss the fundamental point, which is to question the utility of sweeteners in the first place. And it is for that reason that Saccharine was removed from statute as an *"anticipated human carcinogen"* in 2010. Such examples clearly demonstrate the different attitudes of those of us who believe in the precautionary principle and those of us who adhere to notions of acceptable limits, based on sound objective science, and nothing else.

Evidence abounds showing that Saccharin in particular and NNS's, in general, upset the microbiology of the human gut. The consequences include but are not limited to increased blood sugar levels. For instance, research carried out in 2008 found that laboratory rats fed yoghurt sweetened with saccharin gained more weight in the form of fat. The rodents consistently had a more stimulated appetite and so did not shed the extra weight. Equivalent [75] findings have been noted with the fizzy drinks discussed in chapter six. Now, this experiment was one of the first of its kind and you cannot compare the diet of a rodent in a laboratory, with that of a human being in the 21st-century.

However, an apparent identical change in the association the brain makes between sweetness and energy content appears to be driving the altered metabolism. The supposition is that the ingestion of saccharin alters the mechanisms by which the brain regulates sugar metabolism and appetite. However, again it has to be stressed that different people have different experiences, different metabolic tolerances and homeostatic [76] limits. Since 2008 various studies have come to different conclusions, some find evidence of weight loss and some find evidence of weight gain, others are inconclusive. For human studies, the key variable is the diet and any prior consumption of sweeteners. There is huge experimental and statistical variance in any results obtained from these experiments. That does not remove the basic conclusion derived from the subsequent study, which has been continuing since 2008. Experimental data supports the hypothesis that foods sweetened with saccharin and other NNS compounds promotes weight gain and associated syndromes, as compared to eating foods which do not contain them. At the time of writing research continues into both the *"knowing* [77] *it can happen"* and the *"how and why does it happen"*.

## Saccharine Sodium

This section only exists because the Sweetener in question, sodium Saccharine cropped up in the ant-acid concoction a friend uses for his upset stomach. We have all seen Gaviscon or equivalent formulations advertised to treat an *"acid belly"* and they do work in the short term. This particular formulation is composed of a solution of:

- Sodium bicarbonate which is one of three additives designated E 500 1-3 [78].
- Sodium alginate (E 401 [79]) a thickening agent.
- Calcium Carbonate (E 170 [80]), which is ordinary chalk. It has the chemical formula $CaCO_3$ and in nature has a variety forms. As a food additive, it is one of the natural substances we have been using for hundreds of years.

The label then goes on to declare, "It also contains":

- Carbomer [80].
- Sodium hydroxide (NaOH) E 524 [81]
- Saccharine sodium [82]
- Ethyl Para-hydroxy-benzoate (E 214 [83]).
- Propyl *"ditto"* (E 216 [84]).
- Butyl [85] "ditto" ( E ??? hmmmmm)
- Isopropyl alcohol
- Erythrosine Eye colour (E 127 [86] )
- Star anise oil [87]
- Purified Water

A carbomer is a thickening agent normally associated with cosmetics. Sodium Hydroxide is a strong alkali used in many industries. Here it is used as an acidity regulator in that it helps keep the pH of the ant-acid formulation alkali for as long as possible. In 2004 [88] the ethyl, propyl and butyl compounds and their various salts were all declared as safe by the EFSA. However, this does not explain why the butyl form is not listed as having an e number. I have yet to find a sensible reason why this is so; hence I assume the producer does not have to declare it. These compounds belong to a whole class of organic chemicals called the parabens, which are used in cosmetics and over the counter medicines. And this is merely the applications I came across, there will be more. The parabens and their various derivatives serve as anti-fungal preservatives. In the natural world, some are released as behavioural pheromones by pollinating and other insects. The propyl form has been implicated in reduced sperm count in male laboratory rodents. However, a person is more likely to experience an allergic reaction. Generally, the *"parahydroxy"* compounds are not recommended for ingestion by children and some are banned in some countries around the world. Isopropyl alcohol is used in the manufacture of gluten free bread. Presumably, it is used to make gluten free pasta and other food products too. The annual production of isopropyl alcohol is measured in tens of thousands of tonnes. It is used in laboratories, as an industrial solvent, a hydrating and dehydrating agent (a thickener), in household cleaning products, in pharmaceuticals and over the counter medicines. It is even added to liquid combustible fuels where it helps them burn more efficiently and adsorbs some particulates. In food processing, it is used as a flavour enhancer and likely this is one of its functions here. Interestingly it does not have an e number, well not one I could find. The erythrosine [89] is a food and medicine colourant. It is also used in dentistry to discolour any plaque and tartare which may be calling your teeth home. It is also used in hair dyes and lipsticks as well as any other cosmetic product as required and without restriction. The star anise oil is added for extra fragrance and because it has utility in treating stomach cramps. The water is the solution in which all of these substances are dissolved to make the solvent used to treat the upset or acid stomach. Clearly, if you take a look at the ingredients list it seems obvious that a more natural and organic form of the same solution can be made. To that end, my friend is investigating alternatives. However, that is not the reason for this section of text, which only exists due to the presence of sodium saccharine [90] in the solution.

This substance is the sodium salt of saccharine and as an NNS it has a history and controversy [91] which resides in the same dysfunctional ball park as aspartame. In that it is one of those molecules that simply should not be present in any food or substance ingested by organisms, so no change there then! The only reason it exists in the above solution is to add sweetness and mask the real taste of the brew being drunk to treat the stomach upset. I get that totally if you are feeling a bit queasy and vomitus the last thing you want is a liquid that might catch in your throat. It somewhat defeats the object of the exercise does it not? Understandably we all want our medicine to do its job as quickly as possible and ideally without side effects. So, yes, by all means, sweeten your medicine if it means you are going to be able to hold it down. However, I think this draws us to the glaring contradiction with this medicine and it exemplifies totally what I have hopefully imparted throughout this book. My friend is trying to figure out the cause of the stomach upset and so I mentioned a while back the role of NNS's in the diet and the possible impact. I sent him a few links (all of which are in the references) and said take a look and see what you think. He says that he had one of those WTAF moments and stopped taking them straight away. He says that things have improved since he stopped using them and I'm not going to argue. The establishment scientists I have lambasted throughout this book undoubtedly would. After all, this is anecdotal or unscientific and so there couldn't possibly be anything in it could there? Well maybe there is and maybe there isn't, but this is not the point either. My friend still has the upset stomach, but according to him, it is a lot less severe and frequent. He still has his moments and that tells me that NNS's are not the primary cause. They may be intensifying his symptoms or they may have nothing to do with them, they could be acting in tandem with other substances, but it does not look as if the sweeteners are causing his symptoms. Out of curiosity, I asked my friend to send me the ingredients list, the list presented above is the result. Obviously, the sodium saccharine stood out the most, but the other substances were more than worthy of mention too. The conversation went something like this:

**Me:** But this contains SA, I think that's a sweetener

**Him:** What? Really?

**Me:** Hang on a second I'll have a look and get back to you, yup it's definitely a sweetener. I thought I recognised it.

**Him:** Oh, but I want to avoid those, that's not what he said, I can't write what he said, there might be children present.

**Me:** What else is in the ingredients, I reckon there is a section of the book developing here.

**Him:** Well you can only use this story if I get a share of the cash, at which point he started laughing.

**Me:** Cheeky so and so, no seriously, do you mind?

**Him:** No of course not

So here we are then, a situation where a friend is looking to get to the bottom of what ails him so. It could well be that one of the solutions could be contributing. Aside from that when I said what was in the solution he said:

"hang on, most of this just ground chalk, with some other powdered stuff in the water, with some sugar and some pink stuff to make it look better and some sweet stuff there so's I can swallow it without throwing up"

To which I responded "yup, that is about the size of it"

And it was here that the conversation and on his part the research started on how to make his own solutions to deal with or control his gastric problem. From a medicinal perspective, the advice in chapter three is being followed. I think it makes the cross linkages across the various industries and associated concerns clear present and unavoidable if you choose to look.

**Stevia**

Stevia is not an artificial sweetener or indeed a single substance. It denotes the active ingredients in a whole family of approximately 240 individual species which belong to the plant genus Stevia. The genus was discovered in the 16th century by a botanist called Petrus Jacobus Stevus. Stevia has been used globally for over 1500 years, but in the industrialised world, only since the 1970's. According to its proponents, stevia in its whole form has none of the health risks associated with the NNS's. Whole stevia is between 250 and 300 times sweeter than sugar. The sweet taste comes from glucose which is found in active chemicals called steviol glycosides. It is these chemicals that the industry uses and not the stevia plant per se. The glycosides are extracted from the leaves by steeping them in various combinations of acids and/or solvents. [92] The desired active compounds are then further extracted, refined, purified and concentrated. The industry would have you believe that because the active molecules have not been changed during the extraction process, that they are entirely natural. In the US, stevia can be labelled as natural, but not in the EU hence the e number indicated below. The extracted molecules are between 30 and 320 times sweeter than sugar. Up until the early 21st-century in the US Stevia could only be used as a supplement. It was not approved for use as a sugar substitute until very recently. The first commercial application of stevia occurred in 1970's Japan. In Europe stevia is considered an additive [93] and designated as e number 960; it was first approved for use in France in 2011. Very rapidly the rest of the EU followed suit. It gained approval in the US in 2008 and has been on the GRAS (by petition) list since 2009. Well, more precisely the refined derivatives [94] of the raw stevia plant are granted such status, the plant, its seeds or stems are not, which ought to raise the eyebrows of any rational person. After all, human beings have been using the whole stevia plant since about the 6th century and probably before that too. Clearly, something is not quite right. How can it be correct that an active compound from any plant can be *"approved"* as safe but the plant itself cannot be? Well, the simple answer is money and patent law. It suits the manufacturers to have the plant itself deemed unsafe even though it has been used for over 1500 years in its raw form. The industry can more easily profit from marketing compounds the plant contains as opposed to the plant itself. As with additives and food processing in general, stevia is a big global business.[95] From a US perspective, two key players are involved in the production and marketing of Stevia products. One concern is the huge conglomerate Cargill who make a sweetener called Truvia and the other is a company called Merisant who make a substance called Pure Via. The WHO, the FDA and the EFSA all agree that these derivatives from the stevia plant are safe. These compounds are on the GRAS list after the manufacturers lobbied the FDA to petition and not notify (see chapter five) their status. However, the same organisations hold that the same is not true of the stevia plant itself. The industry is in effect saying that all of the artificial sweeteners available are also safe, but the Stevia plant is unsafe.[96] In the disordered world of food processing, the stevia plant itself is not on the GRAS [97] list or equivalent statutes anywhere in the western world. Yet the extracted compounds are and that has to be beyond ridiculous.

The literature explains that the stevia plant contains several active compounds as well as the other compounds which combine to make a plant, well a plant! The natural forms of beneficial plants, spices and herbs do not generally have the problems associated with isolated synthetic ingredients. The main reason being the whole stock of chemicals is ingested. This is not saying that *"natural"* means *"safe"*, far from it. As Chapter five imparts all substances have a toxic limit and that limit will vary between different populations and between individuals. After all, we may all be living under the same sun and under the same sky, but we do have minor (but clear) biological differences, which make some of us more susceptible to a given substance than others. This reality is the fundamental reason why all food additives are tested. The difference between yours truly and the scientists (overall) who are employed by the food industry is that I believe in the precautionary principle, whilst the food industry adopts an acceptable daily intake (ADI) or acceptable limit approach.

One approved active ingredient is a substance called rebaudioside A [98] or reb A for short. Eating Stevia in its natural state leaves a bitter after-taste in the mouth whilst reb A does not. This assertion does not really stand up to scrutiny – that is according to those who have more knowledge on this subject than I. Taste and texture are hugely subjective. I may find whole stevia bitter tasting, you may not. The bitter taste comes from the non-steviol chemicals in the plant, i.e. those which contain no glucose. If you take a second to think about it, this makes sense. If reb A is separated, the rest of the plant is going to have a more bitter taste. Conversely, if the extraction were to go the other way more reb A (or equivalent compounds) would be left behind. There is no sensible reason for this second eventuality not to happen. For mature plants, the relationship is even more pronounced. Either way, would you want to eat a plant that has been immersed in industrial grade solvents and acids? Given a choice I wouldn't and I don't think you would either. So one obvious conclusion presents itself, all of the chatter concerning taste is really an industry sponsored red herring. We are operating in the realm of *"propriety"* and *"patents",* (see chapter two) which means that the Cargill's of this world can profit more from patenting a particular chemical or process, as opposed to the whole stevia plant itself. At its absolute simplest patent law allows any company to take ownership of a particular genetic trait, characteristic, chemical, or biological molecule and then profit from its use as they see fit. So the production of reb A has nothing to do with taste, quality or nutrition but everything to do with generating profits. The sweetener Truvia mentioned above also falls into this category. In late 2008 [99,] The Coca-Cola Company in partnership with the Cargill Corporation began marketing their stevia derivative Truvia. At the same time, a nefariously named operation called *"The Whole Earth Sweetener Company"* through one of its subsidiaries called Merisant began marketing its Stevia derivative Pure Via. On both counts, both the FDA and the manufacturers state that based on sound science these compounds are safe to use by all consumers. Well good for them, but that is enough for me not to use them. Oh and incidentally, I am a human being and citizen of planet Earth; I am not a consumer, no way no how! Such developments mean that compounds derived from the stevia plant are used extensively. Truvia is a blend of Erythritol, Reb A and a selection of natural flavours, whatever that may mean. The point here is that truvia does not contain any Stevia it just contains one derivative, the compound Reb A. Erythritol is the primary ingredient and it is made from corn syrup, which means if it is made in the US it is almost certain to come from genetically engineered corn. Truvia is also coming under scrutiny because it could be exerting the kind of toxic impacts indicated in this chapter. All of the compounds derived from Stevia and used in artificial sweeteners are metabolised at different rates. Reb A, the steviosides and the substances they are blended with, all have different residence times in the body. They will be broken down at slightly different rates in different people. Therefore different people will have different responses or they will have none at all.

The manufacturers are finding the taste of stevia extracts a marketing problem. The Reb A extract gives a strong bitter after taste, similar to liquorice. To compensate for this the manufacturers are engaged in an ongoing drive to mask this taste without compromising the *"natural"* credentials of the extract or the stevia plant itself. The drive is characterised by a whole array of patented (i.e. secret and industry protected) technologies to investigate how the taste response can be altered and manipulated (i.e. made sweeter) *"at a cellular [100]level"*. What this really means is changing the orientation of some of the atoms on the Reb A molecule itself, or substituting them for the atoms of other elements. Here we are talking of the modifications carried out on the various forms of starch discussed in chapter two. A second helpful comparison would be the removal of the three OH groups in sucrose and replacing them with chlorine atoms to make sucralose. The basic structure of the Reb A molecule will not be changed, but the orientation of the atoms which make some of it up will be, and/or some of them will be replaced altogether. According to the manufacturers (Cargill), this will produce *"various beverage applications including carbonated soft drinks and flavoured water that benefit from a natural, reduced calorie product positioning."* It is perhaps little wonder that the natural credentials of stevia based products and the companies which produce and market them have been brought to legal task for their assertions. The bedrock of such litigations [101] is simply that if a product contains extracted or synthetic forms of reb A together with other substances, then it cannot by any reasonable benchmark be considered natural. As a rational human being, it is impossible to disagree. So, you can bet the manufacturers do agree that such substances and the products they contain are natural.[102]

Speaking personally, I believe the manufacturers know the difference between *"natural"* and *"synthetic"*. I believe them to be lying through their back teeth and from the very core of their collective being. On such matters, I believe they perpetuate the lies and deceit to maintain both their position and their profit margin. And make no mistake about it, stevia is big business. For instance, in the US alone the market value for Stevia looks set to approach $565 million a year by 2020, from a base line of some $347 million in 2014. This translates into some 9000 tonnes of raw stevia plant leaf being processed every single year. And that is not pocket money in anyone's language. I wonder how much arable land in the US that ought to be used for growing food has been and will be set aside to grow stevia plants for industrial processing. The money also explains the proclivity for lies and deceit which permeates just through this one section of the global processed food industry. I guess if you have sold your soul on the altar of profit, you are going to want to hold on to the trappings of success by any means necessary. Cargill is not the only player in the Reb A Stevia game but they are arguably the biggest. Other organisations are looking to see how they can alter the structure of a naturally occurring substance in pretty much anyway that they like and then market it as something which it is not. The example of ice cream outlined in chapter three, also demonstrates that such movements are not an isolated instance. In reality, such movements are part and parcel of the processed food industry; they form a core foundation of its very existence. For instance, in 2009 a company called Givaudan began working in the taste alteration arena. This is a Swiss based multi-national who specialises in fragrances, perfumes and cosmetics. If you are wondering why such a company has anything to do with food processing then please do have a look at the section on orange juice in chapter three. The companies' official website is listed below; speaking personally I don't think such organisations should have anything to do with food at all. The industry is looking to develop a whole new range of artificial sweeteners, based on chemicals which can be extracted from the Stevia plant. They are then presumably looking to enhance the *"sweetness"* and remove any residue of *"bitterness"*. Flavour making companies like Givaudan are all too willing to help in this enterprise. By the time any product containing Reb A or any other substance finds its way into your diet, it will have been extracted, purified, chemically altered or otherwise processed to such an extent, that the only similarity it has to the original form is the name. In light of this, our household, when we can afford it, uses organic sugar, honey and syrup to sweeten our culinary creations.

# Chapter Eight: Concluding Points and a Tiny Rant or Two...

It can be argued that if the natural ingredients to make a cake, which would include nuts, butter, flour, berries, cocoa, chocolate, coffee or cream are more expensive than the additives used to substitute them then the industry cannot be blamed. On its own terms, this argument has some leverage. Under capitalism, no profit making enterprise is going to embark in any direction which puts it at a competitive disadvantage. This cold stark reality is referred to as "*the tragedy of the commons*". Until one agency (person or organisation) changes the way it operates and that change bears fruit no movement in any direction will occur. And because any agency that makes the first move has the most to lose no agency will make it. Such are the realities of a world run the way this one is. Within this paradigm, it is to be expected that the "*natural*" will be substituted for the "*artificial*" if it is profitable to do so. If substitution generates profit for organisation A, then other organisations will follow suit. Obviously, this is not the correct direction to embark upon. The tragedy represents one of the many systemic flaws which must be resolved if our species is to have a genuinely sustainable future. If we have a yearly multi-billion dollar business which reduces the quantities of "*natural*" ingredients in the name of "*competition*" or "*confidentiality*" and "*secrecy*" to increase profits, then something has gone very wrong with food manufacturing. Under the current organisational structure the industry will for instance:

- Seek to increase a particular flavour without using the ingredient; it will be an enhancer of one form or another. The enhancers may also serve to mask the taste impact of the addition of extra fat, sugar or salt, and/or the poor quality of the food itself.
- Seek to substitute as many sugars as possible with the

array of artificial sweeteners available, all to state that their product justifies having a *"reduced calorie"* pronouncement.

- Seek to collect and reuse as many different substances and foods as it can from each production run. The lower quality foods and their off-cuts are further refined and processed into ready meals and other convenience foods.
- Employ chemists to calculate how much anti-oxidant can be added to keep a given food *"fresh"* for the longest possible time, within the statutes set out under the law. Legal statutes are under continual attack and subject to change as and when the industry demands it.
- Employ enzymes which provide the illusion of freshness, moistness and palatability thus increasing the shelf life and making a food more attractive for a longer time.
- Use a long life puree, concentrate or gel mixture instead of a fresh fruit or vegetable or any puree you could make from it.
- Prevent food oxidation by coating it with molecule thin bio-films and/or oxide layers.
- Exchange starches for flour and vice versa if it garners benefits of increased volume for a given set of ingredients

Truly, the list of possible alterations and the stated reasons for them is infinite. At any and all opportunities the industry will substitute and exchange where ever it can in the pursuit of maintaining or ideally increasing its profit margin. Any person who believes this not to be the case is not living in the real world. This not to apportion blame, attack or criticise anyone but simply state that as far as food is concerned this is where we are as we approach the end of the second decade of the 21st-century.

For most of us eating some form of processed food is a daily reality of our lives. It is crucial to reiterate that not all processing is *"bad"*. In the absence of some additives, our collective food cupboards would look somewhat different. In addition, it is also absolutely true that some additives are approved for use in both US and EU organic and non-organic foods. For instance, E 392 (alpha-pinene) is the main anti-oxidant extracted from the rosemary herb. However, the organic form will have been extracted directly from the plant, probably by passing steam over it. It will not have been modified either genetically or chemically. If a solvent has been used it will likely be ethanol from a non-GM source. The big food conglomerates can pretty much use which ever solvent they choose. The attitude from the industry never ceases to disgust and frighten me in equal measure. Referring to the "we know better than nature" attitude presented in chapter two this direct quote sums up the attitude of another trade body called the Crop Protection Association (website listed below). On the use of neonicotinoid pesticides (the bumble bee killing chemicals) a spokesman called Nick von Westenholz said in June 2015 (see telegraph reference below) that mistakes made by the organic sector and European Commission recommendations in 2013 *"challenges the perception that organic production is always better for bees and other pollinators, or that a so-called 'natural' solution is always better than a synthetic one".* There you have it in black and white **AGAIN.** They seriously think or project the lie they know better than the web of life which has been evolving for about 3.5 billion years. Both ways, the attitude is absolutely revolting and such people are beneath my contempt. As an associative point when the organic sector makes a mistake in this area, it is quickly rectified and dealt with professionally. All the usual suspects do is throw stones in the glass house and behave like the spoilt petulant children they so clearly are. Yet all of the argument and counter argument around organic and non-organic is irrelevant. They are oxymoronic, to say the least. I do not blame organisations like the soil association for the terminology. They and those who support them have to differentiate from the poison on offer from the big food conglomerates. The organic or intensive food debate misses the

239

point entirely, it is a complete distraction. All food should be produced *"organically"*, whatever the nuts and bolts the word *"organic"* represents. The largely manufactured (pun intended) debate on the need for organic food wilfully ignores one simple reality. The modern *"western diet"* only exists because of technology and its application in food science settings. Yet, the entire industry is largely unaccountable for its actions. We have no real idea as to the life time consequences of the constant ingestion of modern processed foods could be. We are discussing a whole range of negative impacts, from an individual who develops an allergy to full on environmental destruction of entire geographic regions. In the former case how many readers know somebody who has a food or digestive issue? In the latter case, a core driver behind the annihilation of rainforest is palm oil cultivation. The Indonesian Rainforest is on its last legs and I dread to think what will happen when it is finally gone. From an environmental perspective, the whole of South East Asia and Micronesia and Polynesia is in deep and potentially irreversible trouble as it is. Should the last of this once thriving primordial rainforest disappear, what happens next is anyone's guess, but it won't be pretty. The reader can be assured that relatively unspoiled forests, including those in the Congo regions of Central Africa, are next in line. That is if the environmental criminals responsible are **NOT** brought to book for their crimes.

Given a fair and proper choice, most of us would prefer to see additive use kept to an absolute and necessary minimum. The deliberate lack of labelling certainly does not help matters. And it is clear that just because a food may contain 0.6g saturated fat per unit of food, does not mean that the presence of the fat is needed or desirable. The perennial question has to be *"why is the additive present in the first instance?"* And from here you can reasonably ask *"what alternatives are available?"* This point assumes that the label tells you what is really in the food you are buying. Most of the labels on processed foods are filled with deliberately confusing terms, *"spice extract"*, *"fish extract"* or *"firming agent"*, spring to mind. These ambiguous terms are juxtaposed with proclamations of *"high protein content"* or made with *"no added, salt, fat or sugar"*. Even when the name of a compound is stated most of us need to look it up. I have some knowledge of chemistry and know the difference between the different metal salts. Even so, when I saw calcium chloride ($CaCl_2$) I had to check to see what it was doing as an ingredient in a jar of pickled gherkins. This chloride salt of calcium has the e number 509. It functions as an acidity regulator and firming agent for fruits and vegetables. So, again I wonder how long the gherkins have been in the jar. I wonder how squidgy the gherkins would be in the same jar if the calcium chloride were not there. The reader should be asking the same question about every processed food in their larder. I had a quick look at other pickled foods in our cupboards and it is pretty much ubiquitous. It is also used in water purification, as a de-icer and in the treatment of road surfaces. There is no health issue with ingesting the chloride in food; any problems in that department are down to exposure in occupational settings. Having made that clear and taking on board the point being made, to my mind none of this is real labelling. The terms and labelling regime exist to disguise the production method in question, not to inform you as to how the food in question was made.

As I researched and put this book together it became obvious that the issues raised here dovetail with the other bugbear I have repeatedly mentioned throughout my food related writing, which is Genetically Modified Organisms (GMO's) in the human food chain. With that in mind, it seems appropriate to mention them here. The book "Introducing Genetically Modified Organisms GMOs: The History, Research and the TRUTH You're Not Being Told" is an unapologetic, principled and full on broadside attack on:

- The irreversibility of GMO's in the food chain and global environment.

- Where GMO's came from and how they were developed.
- The flat out lies told by the industry which produces it.
- The objectives and machinations of the biotech and life science industry itself.
- The theft of genetic resources by both biotechnology and life science organisations.
- The destruction of objective science and the secrecy of the industry itself.
- The total lack of transparency, honesty or labelling.
- The complete lack of understanding, regard or acknowledgement as to why so many people are concerned, if not downright frightened by what GMO's truly represent.
- The patronising, insulting, superior, flat out racist and arrogant attitudes of those in the scientific community who support it. This corker from a recent forum says it all, *"Imagine the panic of the mass uneducated if they saw the chemical names of benign processing aids."*
- The liars and self-serving criminals in the global political establishment who promote it to your detriment and their profit

The global biotechnology and life science industries would have you believe that genetically engineered crops or animals are exactly the same proposition. They will also state that if I have no problem in principle with the manufacture of enzymes, hormones or medicinal drugs from the activity of engineered microbes, which based on my current knowledge I don't, then I should not be opposed to GMO's. Having said that I think I am going to be somewhat concerned about the use of microbes to make artificial flavours, non-biodegradable plastics or to make specific molecules with specific properties. Why? Well call me old fashioned or behind the times, but I prefer to ingest all the nutrients I need from the food I eat, not in the form of a pill or supplement. I also prefer that food to be fresh in the truest sense of the word and ideally straight from the ground in whole unprocessed form. Returning to the point on biotechnology and to the mention of closed and open systems in chapter two, the manufacture of insulin or chymosin is only possible due to the genetic engineering of bacteria. However, the microbes are kept in giant biological fermenters and there is no contact with the outside world. Clearly, once you plant even just one genetically modified plant there is direct contact and interaction with the environment. The manufacture of insulin represents a closed system whilst planting GM corn, for example, is an interaction with the environment itself. As stated in chapter two the planet is the biggest open system known to us and it is foolhardy in the extreme to suppose that there will not be genetic and therefore evolutionary consequences of planting millions of individual GM seeds of one variety or another. On top of that GM animals or non-food GM crops pose an equal risk of irreversible genetic pollution. I fail to see how genetically modified crops or animals can be seen as a closed system, how can they be? The organism will interact with the environment around it and that means there will inevitably be genetic interactions. No matter how many generations it takes, genes will migrate. And the more generations you have and the more GMO's you have the more gene migration is going to occur. Concurrently, the more unpredictable and therefore potentially dangerous the technology becomes. GM crops and animals are in direct contact with the environment around them. The microbes which produce chymosin or insulin are not. The above two forms of genetic engineering are not the same; they are not even in the same ball park. To treat them as such is at best spurious at worst willingly self-serving and absolutely deceitful. My staunch and absolutely justified opposition to GMO's in food and agriculture does not mean I am anti-scientific. That particular argument from people who support GMO's is the one that really makes my teeth itch. Me? Furious, for being called *"anti-scientific"*, because I happen to give a toss? Absolutely! Calling me or anyone else anti-scientific on that basis is as equally bizarre as calling those of us who oppose the criminal state of Israel anti-Semites, or more colloquially, it is total bullshit.

One has to remember that like all skilled and professional scientists, those employed in the food industry absolutely believe in what they are doing. Equally, their expertise is absolutely essential if we are to ever re-organise the construct known as *"big agriculture"*. Curiously, (and in my recent experience) those who see no problem with additives per se also tend to support plant and animal genetic engineering. It seems the external factors are somehow separate from the constituents of the food in question. I would argue that they are inextricably linked and to say otherwise resides in the house named *"deflection, projection and denial"*. The science is sacrosanct and has established safety, the problem is *"our fault"* and the burden of proof somehow lays with us. For genetic engineering, the science is absolute and infallible and the external (social, political, economic and environmental) factors are irrelevant and inconsequential. In addition, I have lost count of the amount of conversations I have had or seen over the years with individuals (scientists or otherwise) where even when the science is acknowledged as essential (but not enough) the discussion soon descends into mud-slinging and insult, not pleasant, helpful or desirable for anybody. When external factors are mentioned in a discussion on additives, the same attitude seems to emanate from the industry. As far as the processed food industry is concerned once a particular substance has been tested and shown to be safe for use in food processing, there is no issue. Exactly the same seems to hold true from those who support GM crops and animals.

The regulations pertaining to a particular additive are set down and in theory take into account differences in metabolism, individual circumstances of the population who are going to be eating the particular additive. Once it has been approved for use in the EU the substance will be given its own unique E number. The manufacturer can then (if they are obliged to) list the substance as the number and/or by its full name. We are then supposed to trust without question the presence of whichever substances the industry deems safe for us to ingest. One obvious question is to ask *"how these and any other additives might be avoided if they are not fully listed on the label?* How indeed? This question becomes directly relevant when it is remembered that the industry will only list ingredients if it is compelled to do so. The PKU aspect of the story behind aspartame in chapter six is perhaps the most obvious example of this behavior. It is not the only one. Highlighting the dovetail point mentioned above the drivers behind GM foods are as reluctant in 2017 as they have always been to having their product labelled as containing and/or being sourced from GMO's.

The tests for different additives are carried out on animals where the substance in question is mixed into the diet at much higher concentrations than are found in the human diet. The objective is to ascertain whether there are likely to be any negative biological impacts on the population who will be eating the food which contains the additive, i.e. us. The negative biological effects range from the onset of a mild allergic reaction to birth defects or cancer. Other tests are designed to establish if the substance has any real or potential mutagenic properties. A mutagen is any substance or form of energy that causes changes in the genetic code, i.e. DNA. Any changes are called mutations and most but not all have a detrimental effect on the organism in question. In the EU, the results of these tests are assessed and collated by the European Food Safety Authority (EFSA). The data is then used to calculate the acceptable daily intake (ADI) for human consumption. This limit is according to the regulatory authority set with a factor of an extra 100% safety margin. In essence, a daily safety limit is calculated and then this number is divided by 10, then this number is divided by another 10. This is a standard analytical and laboratory technique across the sciences. The ADI is an estimation of the daily concentration or amount of a given substance which can be ingested on a daily basis over the course of a human life span with no noticeable deterioration in health. The ADI is employed by regulatory bodies including the EU, the WHO, EFSA, the UK FSA and the US FDA and through this construct, an additive will be deemed safe or unsafe for human consumption. The ADI concept applies to all people from all walks of life irrespective of age, gender and ethnic group. Once approved the additive in question is monitored and if necessary the status of a given additive is reviewed. The science is only concerned with likely impacts of individual additives. It does not consider the impact of consuming tiny concentrations of many additives over time scales measured over a human life span, (i.e. the cocktail effect). Many thousands of wholly synthetic substances are being consumed on an almost daily basis by billions of people. Nobody can predict with any certainty what the affects really are. Avoidance (if you can) and an adherence and belief in the precautionary principle, would seem to be a sensible strategy. This attitude of establishing *"an acceptable limit"* for substances permeates through the regulatory frameworks of just about every human made substance in existence. A precautionary approach would mean even the slightest possibility of harm would catalyse continual research into less damaging alternatives. The Precautionary principle does not mean framing concerns solely in scientific terms by calling for more research. That plays straight into the hands of the establishment and represents a hoop jumping exercise. A pre-cautionary approach means growing a pair and calling for potentially dangerous substances and practices to be banned, no matter how remote the possibility of harm is.

When it comes to food allergies and intolerances the food industry will attempt by any means at its collective disposal to absolve itself from its own responsibility. As with those who support GMO's the industry will employ the usual mantra of *"a lack of scientific evidence"* or proponents will say there is no *"scientific basis"* and only *"anecdotal evidence"* (read real life consequences) or *"loose associations*" exist. Look at the short section in chapter six and all of chapter three for some examples of this attitude. As far as the industry is concerned any problems are not its fault, therefore the problems are someone else's responsibility, i.e. ours. They will continue to state that there is no real problem with their products. The issue in question is somehow your fault, does not exist, or is caused by other factors. The industry is supremely reluctant to disclose the full scope of its business activities or the additives and other substances it employs. This is why we have wonderful smokescreen phrases which pronounce *"commercial confidentiality"* or *"contractual obligations"*. The industry will continually maintain its alterations and processing activities are carried out for our benefit. These benefits are framed by using words like affordability or convenience and consumer choice. Having said that, one must understand that the industry itself is only one element of the construct we refer to as capitalism. As chapter three imparts the food industry is not going anywhere anytime soon and neither is the wider economic construct it is part of. The issues presented in this book are not going anywhere. On the contrary, they look set to intensify as does the horror which is symptomatic of how things are done, have been done and will continue to be done on this Earth. As far as processed food is concerned the best we can do is make the right choices when we can as best we can on a daily basis, i.e. follow the advice in chapter three. However, be under no illusions the only way things are really going to change for everyone is if the food system itself is as a minimum radically overhauled. That will only happen if we as human beings demand it. And that is that; the end of my third book. Thank you for reading and I'll see you again (so to speak) soon.

# Before you go

Thank you for purchasing my book!

If you found this book interesting and enjoyed reading it, I would really appreciate a short **review on Amazon**. All of your feedback is valuable to me, as your comments and input will be taken on board to help me make this and future books even better.

I would love hearing what you have to say. Please leave me a helpful REVIEW on Amazon.

# Your FREE Gift

Thank you for purchasing this book. To show our appreciation we would like to offer you a copy of our FREE recipe book "BRING LIFE TO YOUR FOOD". To download, visit our website: www.viddapublishing.com.

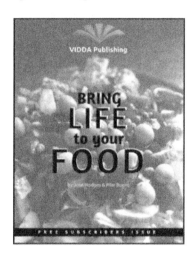

# Free Bonus Chapters: "Food Conspiracy Trilogy"

**INTRODUCING GENETICALLY MODIFIED ORGANISMS GMO'S - The History, Research And The Truth You're Not Being Told** (Food Conspiracy Volume 1)

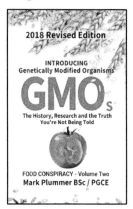

## What to Expect and How To Read This Book

This Book will attempt to provide an objective overview of what genetic engineering (GE) in agriculture and animal husbandry really means. I hope to present a sense of where the science and technology behind GMO's and the drivers behind them comes from and how they are applied. Genetics, GE or GM is a highly complex issue. It connects with science, ethics, politics, international law, human rights, faith and religion as well as social and environmental justice. There is no middle ground with the issue. You either support Genetically Modified Organisms (GMO's) in agriculture, or you don't. To paraphrase Yoda from Star Wars there is no "maybe" or "let's see what happens" there is "support" or there is "not support". The same is true of nuclear power, perpetual war, fracking and climate change, these are red line issues. An individual either accepts a necessity of GMO's in agriculture or they do not. A person supports the rights of indigenous peoples or they don't. You get the point. Either way, it is essential to get some grasp of the principle techniques involved. I have tried to strike a balance between imparting critical knowledge against putting people off by "overdoing" the science, history and politics. It is not necessary to have a detailed understanding of a given technique or be able to argue their respective virtues; this is the domain of those who work as geneticists. You do need to know the nuts and bolts of how GE is conducted. The early chapters contain various YouTube links of the type I have used in the class room. The intent is not to patronise or insult anyone but to advance the necessary biological knowledge. Getting to grips with Genetically Modified (GM) foods requires a basic understanding of how GE is carried out. This book represents only an imperceptible scratch on a very large surface area. There is plenty more research occurring globally in life science and biotechnology laboratories which you, I and everyone else alive today, or in the future, will likely never hear about. This book is an **overview**. It is impossible for **all** the issues raised here to be discussed in forensic detail. So, the text uses real examples as well as hyperlinks and references aplenty by way of compromise and empowerment. As with all non-fiction writing the onus is on the reader to follow up and explore the subject as they see fit. The reader should view the book as a springboard with which to explore subject further. GMO's are **not** an abstract concept or the domain of a science fiction movie. They are real, already here, an irreversible policy and if they really do become the norm, i dread to think as to the future consequences. This writing is at times likely to make you feel uncomfortable, ill at ease or even flat out frightened. This is not my intention, but if you do begin to experience **that** feeling in the pit of your belly, you're eliciting the correct and humane response. The sensible reaction to a policy which is an exceptionally bad idea on **all** counts, a stance I have had since the mid 1990's. With good reason, in 2018, I see absolutely no reason to change my mind. I hope this book will provide a foundation make your **own** mind up on the issue. I will, however, **clearly** state my own position. GMO's in food, agriculture, intensive farming and animal husbandry are not a solution to our current food security problems. GMO's are part of the problem and will only succeed in making matters infinitely worse. Irrespective of other factors, the objectives of the agencies involved in GMO's are highly questionable to say the least. The **only** beneficiaries of the entire enterprise are the transnational corporations and the biotechnology and life science (both defined in chapter three) firms connected to them. This construct is often called "big-agriculture" and is introduced in chapter six. If we are to ever live in a genuinely sustainable world, "big-agriculture" along with other institutions pre-fixed by the word "big" need to be consigned to the dustbin of human history. GMO's have been in our food for about 20 years. They are a product of "big-agriculture" and so ought to be equally untenable. Furthermore, when we know real long-term and sustainable alternatives exist, the stated need for them invites even more questions. GM foods are everything about maximising profits for the biotechnology firms which pursue them along with the agribusiness firms which created and business interests which continue to fund them. In other words, GM foods are last about sustainability, diversity, productivity, or health and nutrition. They are first about profits and astronomical profits too, as well as the control and influence such financial clout brings. I hope the reader adopts a principled position of opposition, but the choice is yours to make and **not** mine to impose.

This book begins with an overview of the history involved with the subject in hand. The middle sections concern how the industry operates and what its objectives are for global agriculture in the future. The last chapter presents GMO's in a frame which stretches back into geologic time. The most relevant period begins at about 12,000 ya. If the reader wishes to they can start their reading with chapter eight, in fact, you may begin your reading at any point. There are plenty of sign posts such as, (see chapter five) or "this point is revisited in....." It is not necessary to read this book sequentially, feel free to navigate as you see fit through the text. Chapter 1 to 4 explain the "how" and "what" of FMO's in agriculture. The "why" is the subject of furious and often vitriolic debate but really comes down (as these things often do) to power, control and money. Chapter 5 will introduce the flavr-savr tomato. The last three chapters will hopefully provide some perspective on the wider economic, scientific and philosophical issues which are intrinsic to a full understanding of GMO's in agriculture. The GM food industry has circumvented the edicts good objective, evidence based science. The industry and its supporters always attempt to rubbish and discredit any science, the scientists or anyone else who challenge its assertions. At its core, this book concludes, aside from generating profits for the industry GMO's serve **no** purpose at all. Furthermore, GMO's represent a technology which has been foisted upon **all** of us based on a pack of **lies**. The same is true of fracking, nuclear power and pretty much any other issue the reader can think of. The middle chapters present a case whereby the whole issue is driven by transnational corporations. These institutions have everything to gain from the uptake of GMO's and plenty to lose should their endeavour fail. The lies themselves are promulgated by the proponents of the technology and an establishment which is in bed with the industry. If I'm being strong here, I ask you to think if the people in charge **and** the politicians who serve them ever tell the truth about anything, exactly, they don't, so why listen to them around GMO's? Transgenic organisms exist for the benefit of the agribusiness oligarch, (see chapter six). They exist as an attempt to gain even more control of the global food supply. GM crops will only exacerbate the very real systemic problems of the current food distribution system. We do not, as of 2018, have the unregulated and unfettered uptake of GMO's in agriculture, but things are looking dicey. If it ever happens they **will** contribute to the global environmental meltdown which is well and truly on the cards, which could result in a total **global** environmental and economic collapse. I hope when you have finished reading, arriving at a **different** conclusion has you swimming in the long river in Egypt, fed by its equally famous tributary without a paddle.

## Do you want to carry on reading?

If so, you can purchase your full copy of "INTRODUCING GENETICALLY MODIFIED ORGANISMS GMOS - THE HISTORY, RESEARCH AND THE TRUTH YOU'RE NOT BEING TOLD" *or the complete "FOOD CONSPIRACY TRILOGY* from www.amazon.com or www.viddapublishing.com

**WHAT HAPPENED TO OUR BREAD? The Chorleywood Bread Process** (Food Conspiracy Volume 2)

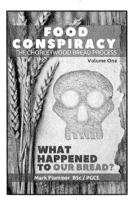

## Introduction

Before writing this book, I knew nothing about baking in 21st century Britain. Intuitively, I knew there were going to be concerns from which questions would emerge. I was not surprised to discover that mass produced bread consumed in the UK is loaded to the max with additives, E numbers and other chemicals. Some of these substances such as vitamin C are familiar to us, others such as mono and di-glycerides, perhaps not. So, if you know nothing about how most bread in 21$^{st}$ century Britain is made, you're in good company. Thus, the principle reason for putting the book together presents itself; very few people seem to know how their bread is made, what it contains or where it comes from. My hope is that this book will go some way to filling that particular knowledge gap. Writing about modern bread making certainly enlightened me; hopefully the same will be true of you, the reader.

First and foremost, this book makes clear that most of the bread made in modern Britain is not fit to be labelled as such. The reason for such a bold statement is simple, mass produced bread can only exist because of how it is produced and the substances added to it. The intention is for this writing to provide a window into the activities of the processed food industry using the humble loaf of bread as a vehicle and signpost to do so. Bread was chosen because it is so familiar to us and is such a staple of the national diet. This book has taken most of 2016 to complete. During that time I have come to understand the degree to which the skill knowledge and experience intrinsic to craft, traditional or artisan baking in the UK has virtually disappeared. Leaving aside notions of food security or self-sufficiency this state of affairs can only be seen as a cultural tragedy. The words *"craft"*, *"artisan"* and *"traditional"* are used interchangeably throughout the text. They are used to delimit the difference between what should be *"normal"* bread and that produced by the Chorleywood Bread Process (CBP). Similarly, phrases such as *"the no time method"* or *"intensive"*, *"mass produced"* and *"industrial-scale bread making"* are equally interchangeable with the CBP acronym. This book presents the case that since the early 1960's the CBP has taken over almost every aspect of

UK bread making. The bottom line, unless you have exclusively eaten only *"artisan"* bread, then you have eaten bread baked by Chorleywood means. When you have finished reading, it will be up to you to decide how you are going to respond. As usual, there will be no preaching or brow beating here, the purpose is to inform and empower. On that note, it is important to mention the final chapter in this writing. Chapter 7 is perhaps the most *"technical"* chapter in this text. It does contain some scientific terms and language that may be unfamiliar. The intent is not to blind or confuse the reader with science. However, a little effort on your part may be required. The intent is again to inform and empower and certainly not to lecture, *"show-off"* or preach. If the reader gets stuck or lost please don't despair. Put the book down (or read another chapter) and come back to it later, with a science dictionary if necessary. It goes without saying that you are free to pose whatever questions you like on the VIDDA Facebook page. Everything written in literature has a purpose and science orientated writing is no different. The scientific concepts discussed are crucial for understanding the science of the CBP. Hopefully, the reader will approach them in the spirit you are intended to.

This book will focus on what the CBP actually is, what actually happens from mixing to baking. The writing seeks to provide an overview of the *"how"*, the *"when"*, as well as the *"why"* of the CBP. Hence there will be no real discussion of sourdough and other forms of bread making. However, plenty of opportunities to investigate such *"real bread making"* techniques and the ingredients used are presented. The research for this book started in early 2016. Within a few weeks, our household was making spelt bread. When a family friend said a bread machine was up for grabs we said: *"yes please"*. It is now gracing us with its presence in our very small kitchen. The idea behind this book is that you will begin to see why and follow suit. In writing this one volume there were innumerable *"WTAF, I didn't know that"* exclamations. This writing will concentrate on the mechanisms, science and economics of modern industrial-scale bread making in the UK. This book is not a novel so you do not have to read it sequentially. As such, feel free to hop around the chapters as you see fit. The writing will attempt to explain how since the industrial revolution bread making has become steadily concentrated and is now under the control of two giant baking conglomerates. That in itself cannot be good for the economic and democratic fabric of the UK. There is no intrinsic problem with the upscaling of production of a given foodstuff or indeed any other *"commodity"*. For me, it is more a question of *"how things are done"* and coming to terms with *"how things are"* and enquiring as to *"how we are going to save ourselves and what is left of the biosphere?"* Having said that, it is counterproductive to hark back to some romantic time in the past, in the land of sunshine and lollipops, where we never grow old and nothing bad ever happens. Such utopian places do not, never have and never will exist. However, this book will attempt to show that the CBP has not delivered the nutritional goods and has been (arguably unintentionally) hugely detrimental to the baking profession and the health of the nation as a whole.

The CBP grew (in part) out of a desire and absolute necessity to improve the food security of the British Isles. The British population was heavily constrained by rationing into the mid-1950's. So, notions of food self-sufficiency would have been given extra attention. The writing will argue that the CBP has morphed from a potentially useful baking technique using home grown wheat into a nutritionally deficient monster, consumed by millions of people every day. Most of whom it has to be said are not aware of what they are eating. I know I wasn't before I started this writing so you're not alone. You would perhaps think that a loaf of bread would fit easily into a definition of *"healthy"*. The objective of this writing is to guide, (with real evidence), the reader toward the opposite conclusion. This book presents the case for wholehearted agreement with what the following quote encapsulates totally: *"bread has been turned from an essential component of a healthy diet to a structure held together by fats, preservatives, emulsifiers and a whole host of additives that have no business being in any food in the first place".*

As an individual, the best you can do to avoid eating CBP bread (and I believe by the end of chapter 7 you will want to), is to invest in a bread machine and learn how to make different forms of bread. If possible the ingredients ought to be purchased from organic, GM free and local suppliers. Dealing with processed food per se requires a total reorganisation and regulation of *"the food industry"* that is not going to happen anytime soon. Such a circumstance will only occur if the industry and those who control it and profit from it are challenged and taken to task head on. This book will impart that the CBP has systematically taken over practically every aspect of bread making in the UK. The writing provides a concise overview of how the CBP came into being and what actually happens in the factory scale bakehouses. The writing will demonstrate that the profit motive has totally subjugated all other concerns. Concurrently, the text will show that bread baked by means of the CBP is the norm and not the exception. In the 21st century, Britain only a tiny proportion of the bread we eat comes from a traditional outlet. I believe this situation needs to be reversed by any and all means necessary. And this book will explain why...

**Do you want to carry on reading?**

***If so, you can purchase your full copy of*** "WHAT HAPPENED TO OUR BREAD? THE CHORLEYWOOD BREAD PROCESS" *or the complete "FOOD CONSPIRACY TRILOGY" from www.amazon.com or www.viddapublishing.com*

# Other Books by VIDDA Publishing

### INTRODUCING GENETICALLY MODIFIED ORGANISMS – GMO's

The History, Research and The TRUTH You're Not Being Told

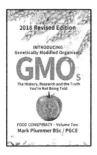

### FOOD CONSPIRACY - WHAT HAPPENED TO OUR BREAD?

The Chorleywood Bread Process

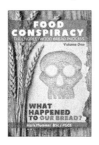

### THE MEDICINE ON YOUR PLATE Series

Understanding Disease, Prevention and Cure with the importance of Plant Based Nutrition and Diet.

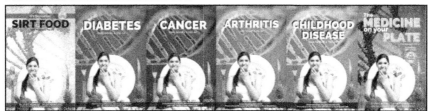

## GREEN UP YOUR LIFE Series

Take control of your health and well-being by introducing Natural, Eco-Friendly habits into your daily routine.

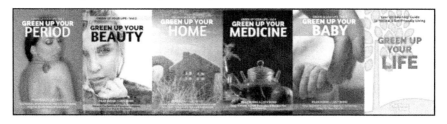

## HEAL YOUR LIFE: Green Lifestyle Trilogy (Nutrition, Lifestyle, Mindfulness Book 1)

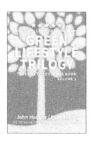

## GREEN LIFESTYLE for WOMEN: Beauty, Period, Baby, Mindfulness

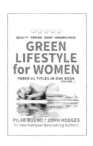

## REEN LIFESTYLE: for Motherhood & Parenting
Healthy Baby - Clean Food - Natural Medicine

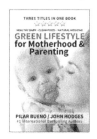

## DOG TALES Series
Stories of Loyalty, Heroism & Devotion

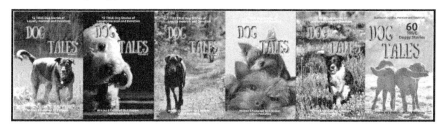

## BUSINESS, INCOME & SOCIAL MEDIA Series
How to Promote, Market & Create Business with Social Media

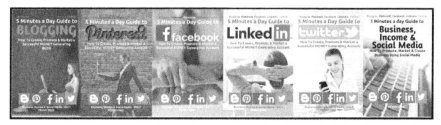

## RESOLUTION TO BE HAPPY
Make yourself smile every day and banish stress and anxiety forever

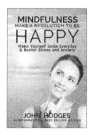

# Connect with VIDDA Publishing

At VIDDA Publishing, we specialise in electronic, audio and printed books in the subjects of Health & Nutrition, Education & Natural History.

Feel free to contact us with any questions or suggestions.

Check out our Catalogue or visit our FREE Video Library.

For your Healthy, Nutritious, Green and Cruelty Free products, equipment and gadgets, visit our online VIDDA Health Stores (US: bit.ly/VIDDAstore & UK: bit.ly/VIDDAstoreUK).

Also, for our favourite supplier of nutrients, sprouting seeds and health products, visit bit.ly/BuyWholeFoodsOnline

Subscribe to our website now and receive a FREE "Bring Life to your Food" Recipe book.

Finally, you can check out our publishing blog "Living like you mean it" for helpful tips, inspiration and updates on new books and free promotions coming soon.

| | |
|---|---|
| Website: | www.viddapublishing.com |
| Blog: | www.viddapublishing.blogspot.co.uk |
| Twitter: | twitter.com/VIDDAPublishing |
| Instagram: | www.instagram.com/viddapublishing |
| Facebook: | www.facebook.com/viddapublishing |
| Health Store - US: | bit.ly/VIDDAstore |
| Health Store - UK: | bit.ly/VIDDAstoreUK |

# About the Author

## *Mark Plummer B.Sc. /PGCE*

Mark Plummer trained and taught science in Spain until a confluence of austerity, divorce and new love brought him back to the UK. He has worked on behalf of most major UK charities, environmental and NGO you can think of. He was a fundraiser, data inputter, administrator and every role in between and back again. Aside from that, he has paid his dues on the chalk face of terrible temporary and agency jobs. Bitter experience has taught him, don't let it grind you down, remember you have rights, join a union and you can say NO!

Today he divides his time between writing, campaigning and teaching. His leisure time involves music, film, literature and the kitchen as well as spending quality time (what other time is there?) with friends and family.

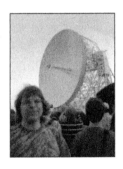

*Mark Plummer suitably attired before Hawkwind at Jodrell Bank Observatory (Summer 2013).*

*For the fans everywhere all over the world: I know it's not Hawkwind but this is a crucial issue... ININHB*

# Sources

## Chapter 1

**Hyperlinks**

1: http://apjcn.nhri.org.tw/server/info/books-phds/books/foodfacts/html/maintext/main2a.html

2: https://www.britannica.com/science/chemical-energy

3: http://www.livestrong.com/article/145529-what-is-cold-pressed-oil/

4: http://www.foodscience-avenue.com/2016/06/chemical-solvent-extraction-in-food.html

5: http://www.ukfoodguide.net/e310.htm

6: http://www.food-info.net/uk/e/e320.htm

7: https://www.britannica.com/science/aromatic-compound

8: https://www.livescience.com/36424-food-additive-bha-butylated-hydroxyanisole.html

9: http://www.sensiblebite.com/2011/07/antioxidants-tbhqe319.html#!/2011/07/antioxidants-tbhqe319.html

10: http://www.chemguide.co.uk/organicprops/phenol/background.html

11: http://www.chem.ucla.edu/~harding/notes/FG_01.pdf

12: http://science.howstuffworks.com/environmental/energy/oil-refining4.htm

13: http://www.chemguide.co.uk/organicprops/alkanes/cracking.html

14: http://www.livestrong.com/article/243789-foods-rich-in-plant-sterols/

15: http://www.heart.org/HEARTORG/Conditions/Cholesterol/HDLLDLTriglycerides/HDL-Good-LDL-Bad-Cholesterol-and-Triglycerides_UCM_305561_Article.jsp#.WT_VZYVOLIV

16: http://www.webmd.com/heart-disease/heart-failure/tc/coenzyme-q10-topic-overview#1

17: https://www.ncbi.nlm.nih.gov/pubmed/23080257

18: http://www.grandviewresearch.com/industry-analysis/coenzyme-q10-coq10-market

19: http://www.webmd.com/vitamins-and-supplements/astaxanthin#1

20: https://www.ncbi.nlm.nih.gov/pubmed/12134711

21: http://www.laleva.cc/food/enumbers/E161-170.html

22: http://www.nutraingredients.com/Suppliers2/Astaxanthin-wins-Novel-Foods-approval

23: https://www.efsa.europa.eu/en/efsajournal/pub/3724

24: https://www.verywell.com/coal-tar-products-for-psoriasis-2788383

25: https://www.efsa.europa.eu/en/efsajournal/pub/4247

26: http://www.food-info.net/uk/e/e300.htm

27: http://www.huffingtonpost.com/2015/03/11/what-is-melatonin-sleep_n_6795220.html

28: https://noshly.com/additive/e322/antioxidant/322/#.WYrQNz6QzIU

29: http://www.sciencedirect.com/science/article/pii/S0927776501001898?via%3Dihub

30: http://www.food-info.net/uk/e/e460.htm

31: http://www.ibtimes.com/mcdonalds-burger-king-taco-bell-more-have-wood-pulp-food-1616514

32: https://qz.com/223742/there-is-a-secret-ingredient-in-your-burgers-wood-pulp/

33: https://www.thestreet.com/story/11012915/2/cellulose-wood-pulp-never-tasted-so-good.html

34: https://www.cybercolloids.net/sites/default/files/E%20numbers%20numerical.pdf

35: http://www.askmarxfoods.com/what-are-hydrocolloids/

36: http://www.cybercolloids.net/news/changing-roles-hydrocolloids-and-food-fibres

37: http://www.cybercolloids.net/information/technical-articles/marine-hydrocolloid-market

38: http://www.realfoods.co.uk/article/how-sulphur-dioxide-is-used-in-food-preservation

39: http://www.food-info.net/uk/e/e220.htm

40: http://www.livestrong.com/article/220542-dangers-of-calcium-disodium-edta/

41: http://www.food-info.net/uk/e/e385.htm

42: http://www.ukfoodguide.net/e160c.htm

43: http://edition.cnn.com/2015/01/14/health/feat-natural-flavors-explained/

44: https://www.efsa.europa.eu/en/efsajournal/pub/2318

45: http://www.food-info.net/uk/e/e516.htm

46: http://www.ukfoodguide.net/e250.htm

## Primary research

https://www.efsa.europa.eu/en/efsajournal/pub/4247

https://www.ncbi.nlm.nih.gov/pmc/articles/PMC1082903/

http://hortsci.ashspublications.org/content/37/2/353.full.pdf

http://onlinelibrary.wiley.com/doi/10.1111/1541-4337.12068/pdf

https://www.ncbi.nlm.nih.gov/pmc/articles/PMC4059325/pdf/bjm-45-49.pdf

https://www.ncbi.nlm.nih.gov/pmc/articles/PMC4411456/pdf/JEPH2015-319727.pdf

https://www.ncbi.nlm.nih.gov/pmc/articles/PMC2669451/pdf/1475-2891-8-16.pdf

## Articles

https://www.britannica.com/print/article/95261

http://www.chemistryexplained.com/Ru-Sp/Salt.html

http://www.chemguide.co.uk/organicprops/phenol/background.html

http://www.precisionnutrition.com/all-about-food-additives

https://www.washingtonpost.com/lifestyle/wellness/not-all-processed-foods-are-bad-for-you-how-theyre-made-matters/2017/02/08/8b205378-ea5b-11e6-bf6f-301b6b443624_story.html?utm_term=.3295a0dd4247

http://articles.mercola.com/sites/articles/archive/2013/02/27/us-food-products.aspx

https://www.britannica.com/print/article/460967

http://edition.cnn.com/2015/01/14/health/feat-natural-flavors-explained/

https://www.scientificamerican.com/article/what-is-the-difference-be-2002-07-29/

http://www.nutraingredients.com/Suppliers2/Astaxanthin-wins-Novel-Foods-approval

http://www.livestrong.com/article/243789-foods-rich-in-plant-sterols/

https://www.thestreet.com/story/11012915/2/cellulose-wood-pulp-never-tasted-so-good.html

http://www.huffingtonpost.com/2015/03/11/what-is-melatonin-sleep_n_6795220.html

https://en.wikipedia.org/wiki/Turgor_pressure

https://qz.com/223742/there-is-a-secret-ingredient-in-your-burgers-wood-pulp/

http://www.ibtimes.com/mcdonalds-burger-king-taco-bell-more-have-wood-pulp-food-1616514

http://www.askmarxfoods.com/what-are-hydrocolloids/

http://phys.org/news/2010-01-chemical-additives-food.html

http://www.organicfoodshq.com/tag/coal-tar/

http://www.huffingtonpost.com/suzy-cohen-rph/astaxanthin_b_2750910.html

https://qz.com/358811/heres-why-your-farmed-salmon-has-color-added-to-it/

http://articles.mercola.com/sites/articles/archive/2010/11/23/astaxanthin-the-eye-antioxidant-550-times-more-powerful-than-vitamin-e.aspx

http://www.cybercolloids.net/news/changing-roles-hydrocolloids-and-food-fibres

http://www.cybercolloids.net/information/technical-articles/marine-hydrocolloid-market

http://www.scienceofcooking.com/science_of_hydrocolloids_in_cooking.htm

http://www.okfoodadd.com/Blog/detail/id/795.html

https://www.acs.org/content/dam/acsorg/education/resources/highschool/chemmatters/archive/chemmatters-oct2015-food-colorings.pdf

http://www.independent.co.uk/life-style/food-and-drink/features/should-we-be-fortifying-foods-with-nutrients-6348759.html

http://www.webmd.com/diet/the-truth-about-seven-common-food-additives

http://www.bbc.co.uk/news/magazine-10773893

https://www.thestreet.com/story/11012915/1/cellulose-wood-pulp-never-tasted-so-good.html

http://www.mnn.com/food/healthy-eating/stories/8-creepy-mystery-ingredients-in-fast-food

http://www.cracked.com/article_19433_the-6-most-horrifying-lies-food-industry-feeding-you.html

http://www.bbc.co.uk/blogs/food/2010/08/are-e-numbers-really-bad-for-y.shtml

http://www.just-food.com/analysis/the-truth-about-coal-tar-in-your-food_id94184.aspx

https://www.food.gov.uk/science/additives

http://healthyeating.sfgate.com/processed-food-definition-2074.html

http://www.nhs.uk/livewell/goodfood/pages/what-are-processed-foods.aspx

http://ag.arizona.edu/pubs/health/foodsafety/az1082.html

http://blog.fooducate.com/2011/08/03/11-types-of-food-additives/

http://hubpages.com/health/Different-Types-Of-Food-Additives

http://hubpages.com/health/Food-Additives-to-Avoid

http://hubpages.com/health/food-additives/2515

https://medicalxpress.com/news/2010-01-chemical-additives-food.html

http://www.independent.co.uk/life-style/health-and-families/features/additives-its-time-to-look-on-the-bright-side-1955043.html

http://saferchemicals.org/2015/02/27/artificial-food-dyes-risky-business/

http://www.foodnavigator.com/Market-Trends/Relief-for-organic-meat-industry-as-EC-calls-off-nitrate-ban

http://www.foodmanufacture.co.uk/Business-News/Soil-Association-seeks-indefinite-delay-on-nitrate-ban

https://www.prevention.com/food/healthy-eating-tips/nitrites-and-nitrates

**Reports and reviews**

http://www.pbrc.edu/training-and-education/pdf/pns/pns_anthocyanins.pdf

http://umm.edu/health/medical/altmed/supplement/coenzyme-q10

http://www.webmd.com/heart-disease/heart-failure/tc/coenzyme-q10-topic-overview#1

http://www.grandviewresearch.com/industry-analysis/coenzyme-q10-coq10-market

http://www.technocheminc.com/oil-refining.htm

https://www.ihs.com/products/chemical-food-additives-scup.html

http://www.chemistryindustry.biz/acidity-regulator.html

http://www.eufic.org/article/en/food-safety-quality/food-additives/expid/basics-food-additives/

http://www.sustainabletable.org/385/additives

http://www.foodmatters.tv/articles-1/dirty-secrets-of-the-food-processing-industry

http://www.fda.gov/downloads/Food/IngredientsPackagingLabeling/ucm094249.pdf

http://www.senseaboutscience.org/pages/food-additives.html

## Industry Web links

https://www.efsa.europa.eu/

http://www.cybercolloids.net/

# Chapter 2

**Hyperlinks**

1: http://www.pbs.org/wgbh/evolution/library/03/2/l_032_02.html

2: https://en.wikipedia.org/wiki/Crossing_the_Rubicon

3: http://www.smithsonianmag.com/science-nature/what-is-the-anthropocene-and-are-we-in-it-164801414/

4: http://www.vrg.org/blog/2010/10/01/glucono-delta-lactone-is-an-all-vegetable-ingredient/

5: https://pubchem.ncbi.nlm.nih.gov/compound/D-gluconic_acid#section=Top

6: https://en.wikipedia.org/wiki/Gluconic_acid

7: https://noshly.com/additive/e575/acidity-regulator-plus/575/#.WXYgcoVOLIV

8: http://www.vrg.org/blog/2010/10/01/glucono-delta-lactone-is-an-all-vegetable-ingredient/

9: http://ukfoodguide.net/e210.htm

10: http://www.dairyconsultant.co.uk/si-cheesemaking.php

11: https://www.ncbi.nlm.nih.gov/pubmed/19075839

12: https://en.wikipedia.org/wiki/Generally_recognized_as_safe

13: http://www.skinstore.com/blog/skincare/gluconolactone/

14: http://www.nature.com/nature/journal/v493/n7433/full/nature11698.html

15: http://www.nature.com/nature/journal/v493/n7433/full/nature11698.html

16: https://www.sciencedaily.com/terms/denaturation_(biochemistry).htm

17: http://www.kmc.dk/kmc-ingredients/kmc-ingredients/kmc-potato-protein

18: http://www.avebe.com/potato-protein/

19: http://www.foodmanufacture.co.uk/Ingredients/Production-starts-at-first-potato-protein-extraction-plant

20: https://www.ground-based.com/blogs/science-research/potato-protein-isolate

21: http://www.foodmanufacture.co.uk/Ingredients/Solanic-unlocks-the-potential-of-the-humble-potato-at-new-plant

22: http://www.petfoodindustry.com/articles/203-protein-from-potatoes?v=preview

23: http://www.bakeryandsnacks.com/Ingredients/Gluten-free-bakery-potential-for-Solanic-s-potato-protein-isolates-after-SA-GRAS-approval

24: http://www.nutraingredients.com/Suppliers2/Potato-protein-targets-sports-nutrition-market

25: http://www.nutraingredients.com/Research/Potato-proteins-offer-blood-pressure-benefits

26: http://www.foodnavigator.com/Science/Sweet-potato-protein-shows-emulsifier-potential

27: http://www.butterbuds.com/faq/index.html

28: https://www.dairygoodness.ca/butter/how-butter-is-made

29: http://cumberlink.com/news/health/ingredient-investigation-what-is-maltodextrin/article_5e08f308-3799-11e4-8d18-0019bb2963f4.html

30: http://journaltimes.com/news/local/butter-buds/article_b10753b4-cd39-5f7d-8266-7ee4d56698d5.html

31: https://www.scientificamerican.com/article/gene-modified-tomatoes-churn-out-healthy-nutrients/

32: http://www.lyckeby.com/en/food-ingredients/products/speciality-starch/microlys

33: https://www.ulprospector.com/en/eu/Food/Detail/5574/349502/Pulpiz-Pulp-Extender

34: http://www.independent.co.uk/arts-entertainment/food-drink-food-for-thought-what-is-modified-starch-1177698.html

35: http://www.food-info.net/uk/e/e1400-1500.htm

36: https://en.wikipedia.org/wiki/Acetylated_distarch_adipate

37: https://pubchem.ncbi.nlm.nih.gov/compound/adipic_acid#section=Top

38: http://www.food-info.net/uk/e/e355.htm

39: http://www.foodmanufacture.co.uk/Ingredients/Starch-sticks-with-non-GM-clean-label-coatings

40: http://www.tateandlyle.com/our-expertise/texturants

41: https://www.food.gov.uk/science/novel/gm/gm-labelling

42: http://www.foodmanufacture.co.uk/Ingredients/National-Starch-keeps-the-pulping-agent-clean

43: http://www.foodnavigator.com/Market-Trends/National-Starch-expands-certified-organic-starch-offerings

44: http://www.ucmp.berkeley.edu/quaternary/pleistocene.php

45:http://www.foodmanufacture.co.uk/Supplements/Food-Ingredients-Health-Nutrition/Simpler-food-labelling-demanded-by-consumers

46: http://medical-dictionary.thefreedictionary.com/Acceptable+risk

47: http://foodconstrued.com/2013/09/carmoisine/

48: http://www.ukfoodguide.net/e122.htm

49: http://ukfoodguide.net/e120.htm

50: http://eol.org/pages/836534/overview

51:http://www.foodnavigator-usa.com/Suppliers2/Rosemary-extract-sees-substantial-growth-in-shelf-extension

52: http://www.foodnavigator.com/Policy/Rosemary-extracts-get-final-EU-approval-for-food-preservation

53: https://en.wikipedia.org/wiki/Carnosic_acid

54: https://www.ncbi.nlm.nih.gov/pubmed/1378672

55: http://www.sciencedirect.com/science/article/pii/S030438351100067X

56: http://onlinelibrary.wiley.com/doi/10.2903/j.efsa.2015.4090/full

57: http://www.food-info.net/uk/e/e300-400.htm

58: http://science.jrank.org/pages/1099/Butylated-Hydroxyanisole.html

59: http://medical-dictionary.thefreedictionary.com/E321

60: https://www.livescience.com/36424-food-additive-bha-butylated-hydroxyanisole.html

61: http://cen.acs.org/articles/93/i8/General-Mills-Remove-Antioxidant-BHT.html

62: https://www.ncbi.nlm.nih.gov/pubmed/20184561

63: https://www.newscientist.com/blogs/culturelab/2012/02/the-yuck-factor-explained.html

64: http://www.scidev.net/global/gm/news/gm-potato-uses-frog-gene-to-resist-pathogens.html

65: http://www.foodnavigator.com/Science/Clean-label-becomes-Europe-wide-trend

66: http://www.foodnavigator.com/Market-Trends/What-do-natural-and-clean-label-mean-anyway

67: http://www.foodmanufacture.co.uk/Ingredients/Clean-label-glaze-cuts-costs-and-extends-shelf-life

68: http://www.food-info.net/uk/e/e920.htm

69: http://www.laleva.cc/food/enumbers/E901-970.html

70: http://www.ajiaminoscience.com/products/manufactured_products/l-amino_acids/L-Cysteine.aspx

71:http://www.vrg.org/blog/2011/03/09/l-cysteine-in-bread-products-still-mostly-sourced-from-human-hair-duck-feathers-hog-hair/

72: http://www.foodnavigator.com/Science/New-technology-for-cysteine-food-ingredient

73: https://www.theguardian.com/commentisfree/2014/sep/07/eating-food-fraud-review-horsemeat-scandal

74: https://munchies.vice.com/en_us/article/53jx5n/theres-human-hair-in-your-bread

75: http://medical-dictionary.thefreedictionary.com/Acceptable+risk

76: http://www.gmoinside.org/substantial-equivalence/

77:https://www.researchgate.net/publication/263970137_Chemical_residues_food_additives_and_natural_toxicants_in_food_-_the_cocktail_effect

78: https://www.ncbi.nlm.nih.gov/pubmed/16352620?dopt=Abstract

79: http://www.bakingbusiness.com/Features/Formulations/2015/12/Permeates-potential.aspx?cck=1

## Primary literature

http://onlinelibrary.wiley.com/doi/10.2903/j.efsa.2011.2392/pdf

http://onlinelibrary.wiley.com/doi/10.2903/j.efsa.2008.721/epdf

http://journals.sagepub.com/doi/abs/10.1080/10915810290096513?url_ver=Z39.88-2003&rfr_id=oripercent3Aridpercent3Acrossref.org&rfr_dat=cr_pubpercent3Dpubmed&

http://world-food.net/download/journals/2011-issue_1/3.pdf

https://ntp.niehs.nih.gov/ntp/roc/content/profiles/butylatedhydroxyanisole.pdf

http://www.viacheminc.com/wp-content/uploads/Product-Data-Sheet-Glucono-delta-Lactone.pdf

http://www.cornucopia.org/wp-content/uploads/2013/02/Carrageenan-Report1.pdf

http://www.fao.org/docrep/w6355e/w6355e00.htm

http://www.efsa.europa.eu/sites/default/files/scientific_output/files/main_documents/721.pdf

**Articles**

https://www.britannica.com/science/Permian-extinction

http://www.theguardian.com/lifeandstyle/2015/feb/21/a-feast-of-engineering-whats-really-in-your-food

http://www.independent.co.uk/life-style/food-and-drink/features/the-great-cheddar-swindle-how-to-spot-a-quality-cheese-from-a-mass-produced-one-8217247.html

https://blog.oup.com/2015/03/artisanal-cheese-chemistry/

http://journaltimes.com/news/local/butter-buds/article_b10753b4-cd39-5f7d-8266-7ee4d56698d5.html

http://ansci.illinois.edu/static/ansc438/Mastitis/control.html

http://articles.mercola.com/sites/articles/archive/2010/12/07/why-is-butter-better.aspx#!

http://gmoinside.org/substantial-equivalence/

http://www.foodnavigator.com/Policy/Rosemary-antioxidants-added-to-organic-additives-list

http://cen.acs.org/articles/92/i6/Extending-Shelf-Life-Natural-Preservatives.html

http://cen.acs.org/articles/93/i8/General-Mills-Remove-Antioxidant-BHT.html

http://www.ewg.org/research/ewg-s-dirty-dozen-guide-food-additives/generally-recognized-as-safe-but-is-it

https://www.truthinaging.com/review/what-is-it-bht

http://cen.acs.org/articles/93/i8/General-Mills-Remove-Antioxidant-BHT.html

http://www.telegraph.co.uk/foodanddrink/foodanddrinkadvice/11458409/From-rosemary-extract-to-sugar-syrup-the-new-food-label-nasties.htmlhttp://www.motherjones.com/blue-marble/2010/03/human-hair-additive-your-food

https://www.theguardian.com/lifeandstyle/wordofmouth/2013/may/13/10-gross-ingredients-food-horsemeat-scandal

http://www.bbc.co.uk/blogs/ethicalman/2009/12/does_your_daily_bread_contain_human_hair.html

http://gmoinside.org/substantial-equivalence/

https://authoritynutrition.com/natural-flavors/

http://news.bbc.co.uk/1/hi/magazine/8753698.stm

http://www.bbc.co.uk/blogs/ethicalman/2009/12/does_your_daily_bread_contain_human_hair.html

http://texascollaborative.org/hildasustaita/modulepercent20files/topic3.htm

http://www.foodinsight.org/Questions_and_Anwers_about_Processing_Aids_Used_in_Modern_Food_Production

http://www.foodmanufacture.co.uk/Ingredients/Clean-label-a-term-on-the-move

http://www.foodmanufacture.co.uk/Supplements/Food-Ingredients-Health-Nutrition/Food-industry-defends-its-clean-label-drive

http://www.foodmanufacture.co.uk/Ingredients/Clean-label-a-term-on-the-move

http://www.foodmanufacture.co.uk/Ingredients/Clean-dream

http://theconversation.com/cocktail-of-chemicals-the-health-impact-of-additives-in-processed-foods-3011

http://www.cracked.com/article_19433_the-6-most-horrifying-lies-food-industry-feeding-you.html

http://www.mnn.com/food/healthy-eating/stories/8-creepy-mystery-ingredients-in-fast-food

http://www.webmd.com/vitamins-and-supplements/edta-uses-and-risks?print=true

https://blogs.scientificamerican.com/food-matters/do-gmo-opponents-have-a-problem-with-cheese/

http://www.foodnavigator.com/Policy/ANH-EU-organic-food-might-not-be-truly-organic

https://en.wikipedia.org/wiki/Paracelsus

https://paleoleap.com/do-people-release-toxins-when-they-lose-weight/

**Reports and reviews**

http://www.westonaprice.org/health-topics/dirty-secrets-of-the-food-processing-industry/

http://www.sustainabletable.org/385/additives

http://www.food-info.net/uk/carbs/starch.htm

http://www.fda.gov/Food/IngredientsPackagingLabeling/GRAS/NoticeInven

tory/ucm361097.htm

http://www.bakingbusiness.com/Features/Formulations/2015/12/Permeates-potential.aspx?cck=1

## Sustainability Websites

http://www.foodforlife.org.uk/

## Industry Websites

http://www.figlobal.com/fieurope/

http://www.figlobal.com/fieurope/exhibit/book-your-stand

http://www.clean-label.de/index.php?page=clean-label

https://www.natureseal.com/

http://www.avebe.com/

http://www.sapharmachem.com/distribution-1/category/solanic

http://www.foodmanufacture.co.uk/

http://www.foodnavigator.com/

http://bbuds.com/food-ingredients/

http://cpack.com/

https://www.natureseal.com/

http://www.ajiaminoscience.com/

# Chapter 3

## Hyperlinks

1: https://www.theguardian.com/housing-network/2016/mar/10/empty-homes-england-scotland-homelessness

2: http://www.mayoclinic.org/healthy-lifestyle/nutrition-and-healthy-eating/expert-answers/monosodium-glutamate/faq-20058196

3: http://www.food-info.net/uk/e/e621.htm

4: https://en.wikipedia.org/wiki/Kikunae_Ikeda

5: https://www.ncbi.nlm.nih.gov/pubmed/22054948

6: https://www.britannica.com/biography/Auguste-Escoffier

7: https://www.ncbi.nlm.nih.gov/pubmed/10736372

8: https://www.newscientist.com/article/dn26854-is-msg-a-silent-killer-or-useful-flavour-booster/

9: https://pubchem.ncbi.nlm.nih.gov/compound/acrylonitrile#section=Top

10: https://www.ncbi.nlm.nih.gov/pubmed/23712097

11: https://www.fda.gov/food/ingredientspackaginglabeling/foodadditivesing redients/ucm328728.htm

12: http://emedicine.medscape.com/article/215100-overview

13: http://www.huffingtonpost.com/2014/12/22/umami-what-is-it-anyway_n_6355960.html

14: http://www.foodnavigator-usa.com/R-D/MSG-Review-dismisses-allergy-concerns

15: http://www.alsa.org/about-als/symptoms.html

16:http://www.bbc.co.uk/schools/gcsebitesize/science/triple_ocr_gateway/t he_living_body/circulatory_systems_cardiac/revision/3/

17: https://www.newscientist.com/article/dn26854-is-msg-a-silent-killer-or-useful-flavour-booster/

18: https://www.theguardian.com/commentisfree/2009/aug/12/msg-allergy-chinese-restaurant-syndrome-myth

19: http://www.phschool.com/science/biology_place/biocoach/biokit/chnop s.html

20: https://en.wikipedia.org/wiki/Goitrogen

21: http://www.greenpeace.org/international/en/campaigns/agriculture/pro blem/Corporations-Control-Our-Food/

## Primary literature

https://academic.oup.com/chemse/article/27/9/843/305859/The-Discovery-of-Umami

https://www.omicsonline.org/epidemiological-studies-of-monosodium-glutamate-and-health-2155-9600.S10-009.pdf

https://www.ncbi.nlm.nih.gov/pmc/articles/PMC3153292/pdf/toxins-02-02289.pdf

## Articles

http://www.bbc.co.uk/news/magazine-34930602

https://www.scientificamerican.com/article/what-is-the-difference-be-2002-07-29/

https://blogs.scientificamerican.com/guest-blog/natural-vs-synthetic-chemicals-is-a-gray-matter/

https://en.wikipedia.org/wiki/3-MCPD

http://www.nhs.uk/conditions/huntingtons-disease/pages/introduction.aspx

https://www.newscientist.com/article/dn26854-is-msg-a-silent-killer-or-useful-flavour-booster/

http://www.smithsonianmag.com/arts-culture/its-the-umami-stupid-why-the-truth-about-msg-is-so-easy-to-swallow-180947626/

https://pubchem.ncbi.nlm.nih.gov/compound/ammonia#section=Top

http://www.foodmanufacture.co.uk/Ingredients/Tuna-trial-a-success

http://www.truthinlabeling.org/III.What%20is%20MSG.html

http://articles.mercola.com/sites/articles/archive/2013/07/15/processed-food-secrets.aspx

http://www.huffingtonpost.com/dr-mercola/msg-is-this-silent-killer_b_491502.html

https://www.theguardian.com/lifeandstyle/2005/jul/10/foodanddrink.features3

http://www.huffingtonpost.co.uk/jonathan-luker/sugar-tax_b_9496014.html

http://www.nytimes.com/2008/03/05/dining/05glute.html?_r=2&pagewanted=1&th&emc=th

http://www.livescience.com/32983-what-are-ingredients-life.html

https://www.food.gov.uk/sites/default/files/natural-toxins-factsheet.pdfAuto1080p

http://www.healthy-eating-politics.com/toxins-in-food.html406p

## Reports and Reviews

http://www.food-info.net/uk/intol/msg.htm

http://www.food-info.net/uk/national/msg-report.htm

# Chapter 4

## Hyperlinks

1: https://www.acs.org/content/acs/en/pressroom/presspacs/2014/acs-presspac-february-12-2014/from-artificial-to-natural-the-food-industry-makes-a-major-shift.html

2: http://www.independent.co.uk/news/business/news/chocolate-bar-20-per-cent-smaller-sugar-reduction-mars-kitkat-dairy-milk-childhood-obesity-a7564131.html

3: http://www.nhs.uk/Conditions/Goitre/Pages/Introduction.aspx

4: http://www.nhs.uk/conditions/Rickets/Pages/Introduction.aspx

5: http://www.food-info.net/uk/e/e330.htm

6: http://www.food-info.net/uk/e/e150.htm

7: http://www.phytochemicals.info/phytochemicals/anthocyanins.php

8: http://www.food-info.net/uk/e/e331.htm

9: http://www.ukfoodguide.net/e211.htm

10: http://www.food-info.net/uk/e/e202.htm

11: http://www.ukfoodguide.net/e954.htm

12: https://www.thoughtco.com/definition-of-salt-604644

13: https://illuminatedhealth.com/concentrated-juices-nutrition/

14: http://www.laleva.cc/food/enumbers/E471-480.html

15: http://www.food-info.net/uk/e/e412.htm

16: http://www.ukfoodguide.net/e401.htm

17: http://www.rsc.org/learn-chemistry/resource/res00000011/gaviscon?cmpid=CMP00000013

18: http://www.food-info.net/uk/e/e401.htm

19: http://www.food-info.net/uk/e/e160b.htm

20: http://naturallysavvy.com/eat/what-is-annatto-a-natural-food-coloring-exposed

21: http://www.sciencedirect.com/science/article/pii/S1631074813003482

22: http://www.fitday.com/fitness-articles/nutrition/healthy-eating/health-benefits-of-tocotrienols.html

23: http://www.webmd.com/heart-disease/ldl-cholesterol-the-bad-cholesterol#1

24: http://www.ukfoodguide.net/e160b.htm

25: http://www.ukfoodguide.net/e102.htm

26: https://www.southampton.ac.uk/psychology/research/impact/food_additives.page

27: https://www.newscientist.com/article/dn2971-food-additives-cause-temper-tantrums/

28: http://www.food-info.net/uk/e/e100.htm

29: http://journals.lww.com/jcge/Fulltext/2009/11000/Annatto_and_IBS.2

7.aspx

30: http://sciencing.com/what-propylene-glycol-5013190.html

31: https://www.atsdr.cdc.gov/substances/toxsubstance.asp?toxid=240

32: https://pubchem.ncbi.nlm.nih.gov/compound/hexane#section=Top

33: http://www.bertuzzi.it/coconut

34: http://www.foodchemadditives.com/applications-uses/2039

35: http://www.food-info.net/uk/e/e525.htm

36: http://treadingmyownpath.com/2014/09/11/why-tetra-paks-arent-green-even-though-theyre-recyclable/

37: https://www.ars.usda.gov/research/publications/publication/?seqNo115=139044

38: https://consumerist.com/2011/07/29/oj-flavor-packs/

39: http://www.toxipedia.org/display/toxipedia/Organophosphates

40: http://www.rsc.org/learn-chemistry/wiki/Substance:Gibberellic_acid

41: https://www.thoughtco.com/six-kingdoms-of-life-373414

42: https://www.ncbi.nlm.nih.gov/pubmed/22368048

43: http://arwill50.blogspot.co.uk/2011/04/ethyl-butyrate.html

44: https://pubchem.ncbi.nlm.nih.gov/compound/ethyl_butyrate#section=Top

45: http://www.ivyroses.com/Define/E220

46: http://www.food-info.net/uk/e/e200.htm

47: http://www.ukfoodguide.net/e290.htm

48: http://www.ukfoodguide.net/e300.htm

49: http://www.ftb.com.hr/index.php/archives/115-volume-36-issue-no-3/857-control-of-enzymatic-browning-of-foods

50: https://en.wikipedia.org/wiki/Diethyl_pyrocarbonate

51: https://noshly.com/additive/e575/acidity-regulator-plus/575/

52: https://www.ncbi.nlm.nih.gov/pubmed/21819649

53: http://www.food-info.net/uk/e/e415.htm

54: http://www.ukfoodguide.net/e415.htm

55: http://www.kikkomanusa.com/foodmanufacturers/products/products_fm_details.php?pf=30107&fam=301

56: http://www.ukfoodguide.net/e296.htm

57: http://www.food-info.net/uk/e/e296.htm

58: http://www.food-info.net/uk/e/e270.htm

59: http://www.ukfoodguide.net/e270.htm

60: http://www.food-info.net/uk/e/e224.htm

61: https://noshly.com/additive/e224/antioxidant-plus/224/

## Primary research

http://www.fao.org/fileadmin/templates/agns/pdf/jecfa/cta/67/annatto.pdf

https://www.ncbi.nlm.nih.gov/pmc/articles/PMC3319130/

## Articles

http://www.kikkomanusa.com/foodmanufacturers/products/products_fm_details.php?pf=30107&fam=301

http://journals.lww.com/jcge/Fulltext/2009/11000/Annatto_and_IBS.27.aspx

https://en.wikipedia.org/wiki/Annatto

https://www.organicfacts.net/health-benefits/seed-and-nut/annatto.html

http://www.ukfoodguide.net/e100.htm

http://www.ukfoodguide.net/e330.htm

https://www.scientificamerican.com/article/experts-why-cut-apples-turn-brown/

http://treadingmyownpath.com/2014/09/11/why-tetra-paks-arent-green-even-though-theyre-recyclable/

http://www.bbc.co.uk/news/health-29986012

http://civileats.com/2009/05/06/freshly-squeezed-the-truth-about-orange-juice-in-boxes/

https://www.theguardian.com/news/2006/nov/21/guardianobituaries.bse

http://www.monbiot.com/2000/11/23/mad-cows-and-manganese/

https://www.britannica.com/science/noble-gas

http://abcnews.go.com/Health/orange-juice-moms-secret-ingredient-worries/story?id=15154617

http://articles.baltimoresun.com/2010-10-17/business/bs-bz-juice-labels-consuming-interest20101017_1_flavor-packs-juice-tropicana

http://www.nytimes.com/2009/01/22/business/22pepsi.html?scp=1&sq=tropicana%20PepsiCo&st=cse

281

https://consumerist.com/2017/02/14/worlds-largest-orange-juice-exporter-producing-excessively-watery-oranges/

http://www.naturalnews.com/034703_orange_juice_flavor_packs_ingredients.html

http://www.nature.com/news/food-preservatives-linked-to-obesity-and-gut-disease-1.16984

https://scienceofrevenue.com/tag/how-tropicana-orange-juice-is-made/

http://www.popsci.com/history-flavors-us-pictorial#page-2

http://www.ukfoodguide.net/e300.htm

https://en.wikipedia.org/wiki/Food_browning

http://www.abc.net.au/news/2016-08-02/avocado-technology-food-processing-crop/7679108?pfmredir=sm

http://produceprocessing.net/article/guacamole-technology-makes-way-for-explosion-in-processed-products/

http://www.oregonlive.com/cooking/2014/10/keeping_avocados_from_turning.html

http://www.authenticcider.com/artisan-cider/

https://www.newscientist.com/article/dn28283-more-than-half-of-european-union-votes-to-ban-growing-gm-crops/

https://thechemco.com/chemical/malic-acid/

**Reports and Reviews**

https://draxe.com/propylene-glycol/

http://www.food-info.net/uk/colour/enzymaticbrowning.htm

http://www.fao.org/AG/ags/agsi/ENZYMEFINAL/Enzymatic%20Browning.htm

http://www.foodmatters.com/article/dirty-secrets-of-the-food-processing-industry

http://www.foodsafetymagazine.com/magazine-archive1/februarymarch-2002/non-thermal-alternative-processing-technologies-for-the-control-of-spoilage-bacteria-in-fruit-juices-and-fruit-based-drinks/

http://www.britishsoftdrinks.com/write/MediaUploads/Publications/BSDA_-_FRUIT_JUICE_GUIDANCE_May_2016.pdf

MECHANICAL PROPERTIES OF ORANGE PEEL AND FRUIT TREATED PRE–HARVEST WITH GIBBERELLIC ACID

https://www.theguardian.com/lifeandstyle/2014/jan/17/how-fruit-juice-health-food-junk-food

https://www.pall.com/pdfs/Food-and-Beverage/FBTBTABFJEN.pdf

http://www.fao.org/3/a-au117e.pdf

**Other web links**

https://www.atsdr.cdc.gov/substances/index.asp

**Industry web links**

https://www.unilever.com/

http://www.tetrapak.com/uk

# Chapter 5

## Hyperlinks

1: https://www.scientificamerican.com/article/only-60-years-of-farming-left-if-soil-degradation-continues/

2: http://www.fwi.co.uk/news/only-100-harvests-left-in-uk-farm-soils-scientists-warn.htm

3: http://medical-dictionary.thefreedictionary.com/Western+diet

4: https://emergency.cdc.gov/agent/strychnine/basics/facts.asp

5: https://pubchem.ncbi.nlm.nih.gov/compound/sulfuric_acid

6: https://en.wikipedia.org/wiki/Lead(II)_chromate

7: https://pubchem.ncbi.nlm.nih.gov/compound/lead_chromate#section=Top

8: http://www.chemspider.com/Chemical-Structure.23302.html

9: https://en.wikipedia.org/wiki/Lead%28II%2CIV%29_oxide

10: https://www.aad.org/public/diseases/itchy-skin/hives

11: https://publicdomainreview.org/collections/a-treatise-on-adulteration-of-food-and-culinary-poisons-1820/

12: https://www.britannica.com/plant/logwood-tree-Haematoxylon-genus#ref225703

13: https://www.nlm.nih.gov/visibleproofs/galleries/biographies/wakley.html

14: http://spartacus-educational.com/chartism.htm

15: https://socialistworker.co.uk/art/10040/The%20Chartists:%20A%20militant%20struggle%20for%20the%20rights%20of%20workers

16: http://www.imdb.com/title/tt0066090/

17: https://www.ncbi.nlm.nih.gov/pmc/articles/PMC1439648/pdf/jrsocmed00230-0104a.pdf

18: http://www.pewtrusts.org/en/research-and-analysis/analysis/2013/08/07/pew-study-details-conflicts-of-interest-in-food-additives-safety-reviews

19: http://www.sciencedirect.com/science/article/pii/0091743573900170

20: http://corg.indiana.edu/delaney-clause

21: http://www.johndclare.net/EC9.htm

22: https://www.britannica.com/topic/European-Coal-and-Steel-Community

23: http://www.food-info.net/uk/e/e420.htm

24: http://www.ukfoodguide.net/e101.htm

25: http://www.livestrong.com/article/254242-what-foods-contain-calcium-sulfate/

26: http://sciencing.com/uses-ammonium-carbonate-8233697.html

27: http://www.okfoodadd.com/Blog/detail/id/795.html

28: http://www.food-info.net/uk/e/e150.htm

29: https://www.businesscompanion.info/printpdf/en/quick-guides/food-and-drink/genetically-modified-foods-qanda

30: http://www.foodnavigator-usa.com/Markets/A-day-at-DDW-The-truth-about-4-MeI-148-years-in-business-150-shades-of-brown-and-a-rainbow-of-natural-colors/(page)/4

31: http://www.food-info.net/uk/e/e500.htm

32: https://en.wikipedia.org/wiki/Trona

33: http://www.food-info.net/uk/e/e440.htm

34: http://www.sciencedirect.com/science/article/pii/0163725893900226

35: http://chemicaloftheday.squarespace.com/todays-chemical/2010/4/26/benzoic-acid.html

36: http://news.bbc.co.uk/1/hi/health/4465871.stm

37: https://www.britannica.com/science/saltpeter

38: http://www.ukfoodguide.net/e252.htm

39: http://www.ukfoodguide.net/e249.htm

40: http://www.foodborneillness.com/botulism_food_poisoning/

41: http://www.sciencemuseum.org.uk/broughttolife/people/paracelsus

42: https://www.britannica.com/science/homeostasis

43: https://www.ncbi.nlm.nih.gov/pubmed/15212220

44: https://consumerist.com/2016/03/29/campbell-soup-company-will-switch-to-all-bpa-free-packaging-by-2017/

45: http://www.businesswire.com/news/home/20160329006083/en/Del-Monte-Foods-Announces-Conversion-Non-BPA-Packaging

46: http://ajcn.nutrition.org/content/46/1/201.short?cited-by=yes&legid=ajcn;46/1/201

**Primary Research**

http://ajcn.nutrition.org/content/81/2/341.full.pdf+html

## Articles

https://en.wikipedia.org/wiki/Gypsum

https://en.wikipedia.org/wiki/Copper(II)_sulfate

http://www.huffingtonpost.com/2014/10/03/salicylic-acid-skincare_n_5919712.html

https://en.wikipedia.org/wiki/Borax

http://www.history.com/news/hungry-history/food-fraud-a-brief-history-of-the-adulteration-of-food

https://en.wikipedia.org/wiki/Western_pattern_diet

http://www.livestrong.com/article/111493-foods-contain-salicylic-acid/

http://www.webmd.com/allergies/salicylate-allergy

https://www.chemistryworld.com/podcasts/borax/8250.article

https://www.cancer.org/cancer/cancer-causes/formaldehyde.html

http://spartacus-educational.com/PRwakely.htm

http://www.history.com/news/remembering-the-wounded-knee-massacre

http://www.fooddive.com/news/what-will-the-trump-administration-mean-for-the-food-industry/434085/

https://www.vox.com/2017/4/29/15479488/donald-trump-michelle-obama-school-lunch-menu-labels

http://www.cfs.gov.hk/english/multimedia/multimedia_pub/multimedia_pub_fsf_42_01.html

http://www.esquire.com/food-drink/food/a23169/poison-squad/

http://www.atlasobscura.com/articles/food-testing-in-1902-featured-a-tuxedoclad-poison-squad-eating-plates-of-acid

http://www.mnn.com/food/healthy-eating/stories/whats-the-difference-between-nitrates-and-nitrites

http://www.independent.co.uk/life-style/health-and-families/features/additives-its-time-to-look-on-the-bright-side-1955043.html

http://www.nhs.uk/Conditions/cosmetic-treatments-guide/Pages/botulinum-toxin-Botox-injections.aspx

http://www.greenbiologics.com/blog/what-are-clostridia/

http://www.encyclopedia.com/science-and-technology/biology-and-genetics/cell-biology/sporulation

http://jamanetwork.com/journals/jamainternalmedicine/fullarticle/1725123

https://www.theguardian.com/sustainable-business/2016/mar/31/bpa-chemical-canned-food-general-mills-campbells-soup-del-monte-fda

https://www.sciencedaily.com/releases/2016/02/160201103543.htm

http://www.sciencedaily.com/releases/2011/10/111026122404.htm

http://www.monbiot.com/2015/03/25/3703/

http://www.feednavigator.com/Regulation/Unauthorized-GM-Bacillus-subtilis-production-strain-identified-in-a-vitamin-B2-feed-additive

http://www.sciencedaily.com/releases/2014/11/141116094228.htm

http://www.huffingtonpost.com/alison-brown-ms/food-additives_b_3863317.html

http://www.npr.org/sections/thesalt/2015/04/14/399591292/why-the-fda-is-clueless-about-some-of-the-additives-in-our-food

http://www.preparedfoods.com/articles/103746-gras-ingredients-in-the-21st-century

https://www.nrdc.org/sites/default/files/safety-loophole-for-chemicals-in-food-report.pdf

http://tongsofficial.com/health/generally-recognized-as-safe-gras-what-is-it/

http://federal.laws.com/meat-inspection-act
http://articles.mercola.com/sites/articles/archive/2013/03/21/addictive-junk-food.aspx

http://articles.mercola.com/sites/articles/archive/2013/03/17/senomyx-flavor-enhancers.aspx

https://eic.rsc.org/section/feature/the-fight-against-food-adulteration/2020253.article

http://foodadditive.blogspot.co.uk/2010/12/history-of-food-additive.html

http://www.world-foodhistory.com/2010/02/modern-history-of-food-additives.html

http://www.bbc.co.uk/blogs/food/2010/08/are-e-numbers-really-bad-for-y.shtml

**Reports and reviews**

http://www.pewtrusts.org/~/media/legacy/uploadedfiles/phg/content_level_pages/reports/foodadditivescapstonereportpdf.pdf

http://jamanetwork.com/journals/jamainternalmedicine/fullarticle/1725123

http://www.foodprocessing.com/articles/2010/colorants/

http://www.westonaprice.org/health-topics/dirty-secrets-of-the-food-processing-industry/

http://www.fedup.com.au/factsheets/additive-and-natural-chemical-factsheets/249-252-nitrates-nitrites-and-nitrosamines

http://www.who.int/mediacentre/factsheets/fs270/en/

# Chapter 6

## Hyperlinks

1: http://www.ucmp.berkeley.edu/precambrian/archean_hadean.php

2: http://ideas.time.com/2013/02/05/can-we-drink-soda-responsibly/

3: https://www.theguardian.com/world/shortcuts/2015/apr/28/diet-pepsi-dropped-aspatame-in-us-is-artificial-sweetener-dangerous

4: http://money.cnn.com/2015/08/10/news/companies/diet-pepsi-no-aspartame/

5: http://www.bbc.co.uk/news/health-32478203

6: http://www.forbes.com/sites/greatspeculations/2015/05/21/what-could-removing-aspartame-from-diet-pepsi-do-for-pepsico/#2715e4857a0b4ae011652273

7: http://www.nhs.uk/Livewell/Goodfood/Pages/the-truth-about-acesulfame-k.aspx

8: http://www.ukfoodguide.net/e950.htm

9: http://www.foodnavigator-usa.com/Suppliers2/New-sweetener-to-hit-market-hungry-for-alternatives

10: https://en.wikipedia.org/wiki/Dichloromethane

11: http://www.euractiv.com/section/agriculture-food/news/scientists-once-again-question-the-safety-of-aspartame/

12: http://www.efsa.europa.eu/en/topics/topic/aspartame

13: http://static.diabetesselfmanagement.com/pdfs/DSM0310_012.pdf

14: http://www.independent.co.uk/news/worlds-top-sweetener-is-made-with-gm-bacteria-1101176.html

15: https://www.ncbi.nlm.nih.gov/pubmed/22385158

16: http://www.bloomberg.com/research/stocks/private/snapshot.asp?privcapid=686333

17: https://www.forbes.com/sites/matthewherper/2014/03/12/heres-how-big-pfizer-is/#51b93a281c6e

18: https://pubchem.ncbi.nlm.nih.gov/compound/aspartame#section=Top

19: http://www.biology.arizona.edu/biochemistry/problem_sets/aa/aspartate.html

20: http://www.livestrong.com/article/389334-a-list-of-foods-containing-aspartame/

21: https://supersweetblog.wordpress.com/list-of-products-containing-aspartame/

22: http://www.md-health.com/What-Foods-Contain-Aspartame.html

23: https://www.britannica.com/science/methanol

24: http://www.differencebetween.net/science/difference-between-ethanol-and-methanol/

25: https://www.britannica.com/science/formic-acid

26: https://www.ncbi.nlm.nih.gov/pubmed/23553132

27: http://thebrain.mcgill.ca/flash/i/i_01/i_01_m/i_01_m_ana/i_01_m_ana.html

28: https://www.psychologytoday.com/blog/mouse-man/200904/what-is-dopamine

29: http://undsci.berkeley.edu/article/howscienceworks_16

30: https://www.theguardian.com/notesandqueries/query/0,5753,-2901,00.html

31: https://www.ncbi.nlm.nih.gov/pubmed/8939194

32: https://www.ncbi.nlm.nih.gov/pubmed/23553132

33:https://www.fda.gov/food/ingredientspackaginglabeling/foodadditivesingredients/ucm208580.htm

34: http://www.digitaljournal.com/article/325859

35: https://socialistworker.co.uk/public/searchByCategory/14?searchTitle=The+Troublemaker

36: https://www.sciencedaily.com/releases/2014/01/140116162010.htm

37: http://www.gao.gov/products/HRD-87-46

38: http://www.nspku.org/information/whatispku

39: https://ghr.nlm.nih.gov/gene/PAH#sourcesforpage

40: http://chemistry.elmhurst.edu/vchembook/635pku.html

41: http://pkuadults.tripod.com/id13.html

42: https://www.ncbi.nlm.nih.gov/pubmed/23553132

43: http://www.nhs.uk/conditions/Fibromyalgia/pages/introduction.aspx

44: http://www.independent.co.uk/life-style/health-and-families/diet-fizzy-drinks-dementia-strokes-triple-risk-study-boston-university-a7694421.html

45: https://medlineplus.gov/ency/article/000335.htm

46: https://www.ncbi.nlm.nih.gov/pubmed/22457081

47: http://www.jameslavin.com/articles/2010/08/05/thanks-for-the-brain-cancer-rumsfeld-and-reagan/

48:https://news.google.com/newspapers?id=YvMPAAAAIBAJ&sjid=yYwDA
AAAIBAJ&dq=searle+grand-
jury+fraud+aspartame&pg=5988,2630396&hl=en

49: http://statelaws.findlaw.com/criminal-laws/details-on-state-criminal-statute-of-limitations.html

50: http://www.stltoday.com/news/local/obituaries/dr-john-w-olney-pioneering-brain-scientist/article_f5d6f2b2-d568-5be9-acdd-2187c319e0c0.html

51: http://www.sweetpoison.com/articles/0706/fda_decision_of_the_publi.
html

52: https://www.ucsf.edu/news/2007/01/7408/former-pharmacy-dean-and-head-fda-jere-goyan-has-died

53: http://www.upi.com/Archives/1980/11/22/Members-of-Ronald-Reagans-transition-team-say-their-first/1139343717200/

54: http://www.nytimes.com/2010/03/01/health/policy/01hayes.html

55: http://www.naturalnewsblogs.com/avoiding-aspartame-will-save-health-life/

56: http://www.nndb.com/people/194/000130801/

57: https://monsanto.com/company/history/articles/former-monsanto-products/

58: http://www.independent.co.uk/news/world/3-things-we-know-about-the-secretive-bilderberg-group-and-1-thing-well-never-know-10307054.html

59: http://www.nytimes.com/1985/07/19/business/monsanto-to-acquire-g-d-searle.html

60: http://www4.dr-rath-foundation.org/open_letters/rumsfeld.htm

61: http://www.nbcnews.com/tech/video-games/donald-rumsfeld-launches-churchill-solitaire-gaming-app-n503556

62: http://www.digitaljournal.com/article/336384

63:http://www.mintel.com/press-centre/food-and-drink/stevia-set-to-steal-intense-sweetener-market-share-by-2017-reports-mintel-and-leatherhead-food-research

## Primary Research

http://www.tandfonline.com/doi/pdf/10.3109/01480545.2012.658403?needAccess=true

https://www.researchgate.net/publication/279712596_Aspartame_Methanol_and_the_public_health

http://www.pnas.org/content/106/12/4894.full.pdf

http://jnen.oxfordjournals.org/content/jnen/55/11/1115.full.pdf

http://www.termedia.pl/Review-paper-Effects-of-aspartame-metabolites-on-astrocytes-and-neurons,20,20489,1,1.html

http://www.lightenyourtoxicload.com/wp-content/uploads/2014/07/Dr-Walton-survey-of-aspartame-studies.pdf

https://www.ncbi.nlm.nih.gov/pmc/articles/PMC3953764/pdf/AJPH.2013.301556.pdf

http://while-science-sleeps.com/pdf/211.pdf

https://www.researchgate.net/publication/269637605_Diet_Drink_Consumption_and_the_Risk_of_Cardiovascular_Events_A_Report_from_the_Women%27s_Health_Initiative

http://ajcn.nutrition.org/content/early/2012/10/23/ajcn.111.030833.full.pdf+html

## Articles

http://chemicalsareyourfriends.com/posts/synthetic-sweeteners-chemicals-that-are-finger-lickin-sweet/

http://www.britannica.com/topic/soft-drink

http://www.newworldencyclopedia.org/entry/Methanol

http://www.bbc.co.uk/news/magazine-35461270

http://umm.edu/health/medical/altmed/supplement/phenylalanine

http://www.sourcewatch.org/index.php/Aspartame

http://chemistry.elmhurst.edu/vchembook/549aspartame.html

http://www.madehow.com/Volume-3/Aspartame.html

https://scienceaid.net/chemistry/organic/alcohols.html

http://www.collective-evolution.com/2015/06/09/the-end-of-diet-soda-huge-study-links-aspartame-to-these-major-health-problems/

http://mediaroots.org/bitter-sweetener/

https://www.chemistryworld.com/podcast/aspartame/8068.article

http://www.unionsafety.eu/docs/CoordReports/WorldsMostPopularArtificial
SweetenerRebrandedAsCancerClaimsContinueSpecialReport.html

https://www.sott.net/article/125706-Nations-starting-to-Ban-Aspartame

http://www.drugsdb.com/cib/aspartame/medications-that-contain-
aspartame/
http://www.cdc.gov/mmwr/preview/mmwrhtml/00000426.htm
http://www.cdc.gov/niosh/docs/81-111/

http://emedicine.medscape.com/article/1174890-overview

http://www.huffingtonpost.com/dr-mercola/aspartame-health-
risks_b_668692.html

https://www.honeycolony.com/article/excitotoxins-the-fda-approved-way-
to-damage-your-brain/

http://donellameadows.org/archives/farewell-to-the-delaney-amendment/

http://www.collective-evolution.com/2012/10/06/aspartame-damages-the-
brain-at-any-dose/

http://criminal.findlaw.com/criminal-law-basics/time-limits-for-charges-
state-criminal-statutes-of-limitations.html

https://now.uiowa.edu/2014/03/ui-study-finds-diet-drinks-associated-heart-
trouble-older-women

https://www.sott.net/article/149206-Dr-John-Olney-on-Brain-tumors-and-
aspartame

http://www.nhs.uk/conditions/phenylketonuria/Pages/Introduction.aspx

http://www.uabmedicine.org/news/Food+%28sugar+substitutes%29
http://www.mpwhi.com/aspartame_methanol_and_public_health.pdf
http://www.ncbi.nlm.nih.gov/pubmed/22385158

http://www.huffingtonpost.com/robbie-gennet/donald-rumsfeld-and-the-
s_b_805581.html

http://www.rense.com/general33/legal.htm

http://www.nature.com/scitable/topicpage/mendelian-genetics-patterns-of-
inheritance-and-single-
966https://www.sciencedaily.com/releases/2011/06/110627183944.htm

http://www.scientificamerican.com/article/artificial-sweeteners-may-change-
our-gut-bacteria-in-dangerous-ways/

http://articles.mercola.com/sites/articles/archive/2011/08/03/just-how-bad-
is-aspartame.aspx

http://www.theguardian.com/lifeandstyle/2013/aug/04/demon-drink-war-on-sugar

https://www.drugs.com/coumadin.html

https://en.wikipedia.org/wiki/Phenylalanine_hydroxylase

https://en.wikipedia.org/wiki/Phenylketonuria

https://now.uiowa.edu/2014/03/ui-study-finds-diet-drinks-associated-heart-trouble-older-women

http://www.mpwhi.com/fda_admits_aspartme_causes_birth_defects.htm

http://www.independent.co.uk/life-style/health-and-families/what-is-lupus-what-are-the-symptoms-and-is-treatment-readily-available-a6686246.html

https://www.sciencebasedmedicine.org/aspartame-truth-vs-fiction/

http://www.andeal.org/topic.cfm?cat=4089

 http://www.scoop.co.nz/stories/WO1102/S00839/courageous-fda-whistleblower-jerome-bressler-died.htm

http://www.healthcare.uiowa.edu/alumni/interviews/olney_john.html

http://traitor666.blogspot.co.uk/2006/05/aspartame-donalds-very-own-wmd.html

http://www.collective-evolution.com/2013/01/19/the-shocking-story-of-how-aspartame-became-legal/

http://www.nytimes.com/1989/11/19/business/nutrasweet-s-bitter-fight.html?pagewanted=all

http://www.collective-evolution.com/2012/12/09/aspartame-linked-leukemia-lymphoma-groundbreaking-study/

http://www.organicfoodshq.com/aspartame-natural-sweetener/

http://articles.mercola.com/sites/articles/archive/2009/01/10/aspartame-brain-cancer-and-the-fda.aspx

http://whatreallyhappened.com/WRHARTICLES/fdahidaspartamedata.php

http://therawreport.org/tag/dr-john-olney/

http://mrhoyestokwebsite.com/WOKs/Perception/Related%20Articles/Tricking%20Your%20Tastebuds.pdf

http://www.rense.com/general80/rec.htm

http://www.laleva.org/eng/2004/09/aspartame_poisoning_millions_betty_martini.

http://www.rense.com/general96/aspardeath.html

## Reports

http://archive.gao.gov/d4t4/130780.pdf

http://www.dorway.com/raoreport.pdf

http://www.hc-sc.gc.ca/fn-an/securit/addit/sweeten-edulcor/aspartame-eng.php

http://www.euractiv.com/section/health-consumers/news/eu-food-safety-agency-says-aspartame-poses-no-risk-for-consumers/

http://www.mpwhi.com/thomas_f_x_collins_file.pdf

http://www.arizonaadvancedmedicine.com/Articles/2013/June/Aspartame-History-of-Getting-FDA-Approval.aspx

http://www.efsa.europa.eu/en/topics/topic/aspartame

http://www.nhs.uk/news/2015/03March/Pages/Research-casts-doubt-on-aspartame-sensitivity.aspx

http://www.mpwhi.com/fda_admits_aspartme_causes_birth_defects.htm

http://www.thelupussite.com/practical_information/aspartame.html

http://www.whatreallyhappened.com/WRHARTICLES/fdahidaspartamedata.phphttp://www.mpwhi.com/complete_bressler_report.pdf

http://www.mercola.com/article/aspartame/fraud.htm

http://www.mpwhi.com/thomas_f_x_collins_file.pdf

http://www.wnho.net/letter_to_fda_aspartame_and_free_methyl_alcohol.htm

http://www.sourcewatch.org/index.php/Aspartame

http://www.wnho.net/aspartame_and_children_report.htm

https://dash.harvard.edu/bitstream/handle/1/8846759/Nill,_Ashley_-_The_History_of_Aspartame.pdf?sequence=3

http://www.lightenyourtoxicload.com/wp-content/uploads/2014/07/Dr-Walton-survey-of-aspartame-studies.pdf

http://www.wnho.net/aspartame_and_children_report.htm

http://www.thetruthaboutstuff.com/review1.html

http://www.mpwhi.com/aspartame_methanol_and_public_health.pdf

http://www.dorway.com/thetoxins.html

https://medium.com/@DonRumsfeld/at-83-i-decided-to-develop-an-app-dadd4e53d342

**Related websites**

https://www.cdc.gov/

http://www.mercola.com/forms/background.htm

**Industry web sites**

https://aspartame.org/aspartame-products/

http://bilderbergmeetings.org/

# Chapter 7

**Hyperlinks**

1: http://www.livestrong.com/article/464851-why-is-high-fructose-corn-syrup-banned-in-europe/

2: https://pubchem.ncbi.nlm.nih.gov/compound/D-fructose#section=Top

3: http://www.orthomolecular.org/nutrients/mono.html

4: https://www.ncbi.nlm.nih.gov/pmc/articles/PMC239444/

5: http://www.huffingtonpost.com/dr-mark-hyman/high-fructose-corn-syrup_b_4256220.html

6: http://www.mayoclinic.org/diseases-conditions/nonalcoholic-fatty-liver-disease/home/ovc-20211638

7: https://gmoanswers.com/ask/does-high-fructose-corn-syrup-contain-gmos

8: https://www.statista.com/statistics/249681/total-consumption-of-sugar-worldwide/

9: https://www.theguardian.com/world/2004/aug/12/foodanddrink

10: http://www.nytimes.com/2011/06/17/world/europe/17copenhagen.html

11: http://www.bbc.co.uk/schools/gcsebitesize/science/21c/life_on_earth/species_interdependencerev6.shtml

12: https://www.researchgate.net/publication/250084551_The_Global_Phosphorus_Cycle_Past_Present_and_Future

13: http://www.telegraph.co.uk/finance/newsbysector/retailandconsumer/7866357/Tate-and-Lyle-bids-farewell-to-historic-sugar-and-golden-syrup-business.html

14: http://www.livestrong.com/article/274155-what-is-dextrose-in-food/

15: http://www.food-info.net/uk/glossary/g.htm#glucose

16: http://www.livestrong.com/article/502241-the-risks-of-maltodextrin/

17: http://www.livestrong.com/article/534228-glucose-vs-dextrose/

18: https://en.wikipedia.org/wiki/Maltodextrin

19: http://ic.steadyhealth.com/sucralose-side-effects-and-warnings

20: http://www.ukfoodguide.net/e420.htm

21: http://www.food-info.net/uk/e/e420.htm

22: http://www.nhs.uk/Livewell/Goodfood/Pages/the-truth-about-sucralose.aspx

23: http://www.sugar-and-sweetener-guide.com/e-number-index-for-sweeteners.html

24: http://www.joslin.org/info/what_are_sugar_alcohols.html

25: http://juicingtherainbow.com/671/supermarket-juices/erythritol-e968/

26: http://www.food-info.net/uk/e/e422.htm

27: http://www.ukfoodguide.net/e953.htm

28: http://www.ivyroses.com/Define/E953

29: https://en.wikipedia.org/wiki/Lactitol

30: http://www.food-info.net/uk/e/e966.htm

31: http://www.food-info.net/uk/e/e421.htm

32: http://www.ivyroses.com/Define/E421

33: http://www.ivyroses.com/Define/E967

34: http://www.food-info.net/uk/e/e967.htm

35: https://en.wikipedia.org/wiki/Xylan

36: http://www.huffingtonpost.co.uk/Jenna-Downes/aspartame-sweetener_b_11349520.html

37: https://www.ncbi.nlm.nih.gov/pubmed/8234920

38: https://www.ncbi.nlm.nih.gov/pubmed/18535548

39: https://www.ncbi.nlm.nih.gov/pubmed/3714671?dopt=Abstract

40: http://www.nature.com/nature/journal/v514/n7521/full/nature13793.html

41: https://en.wikipedia.org/wiki/Glycogenesis

42: https://www.sciencedaily.com/releases/2013/12/131218095359.htm

43: https://entomology.ca.uky.edu/ef621

44: https://en.wikipedia.org/wiki/Mesolimbic_pathway

45: http://www.nature.com/nature/journal/v535/n7611/full/535203e.html

46: https://www.ncbi.nlm.nih.gov/pubmed/17212793

47: https://www.ncbi.nlm.nih.gov/pubmed/17693746

48: https://www.psychologytoday.com/basics/dopamine

49: https://www.theguardian.com/public-leaders-network/2011/apr/28/school-food-revolution-threat-cuts

50: https://www.biglotteryfund.org.uk/global-content/press-releases/uk-wide/220217_uk_soil_association_receives_1_25_million_funding_improve_food_older_people

51: http://www.prevention.com/food/healthy-eating-tips/health-risks-sucralose

52: https://www.sciencedaily.com/releases/2014/03/140310111315.htm

53: https://www.ncbi.nlm.nih.gov/pubmed/23712097

54: http://www.sciencedirect.com/science/article/pii/S0273230009000786

55: http://www.sciencedirect.com/science/article/pii/S0278691500000351?np=y

56: http://www.urbandictionary.com/define.php?term=j%27accuse

57: http://www.toxipedia.org/display/toxipedia/Phosgene

58: https://www.livescience.com/39248-what-is-mustard-gas.html

59: https://webhost.bridgew.edu/jhayesboh/TRIPS/EAGLES/FACTS_ABOUT_DDT.htm

60: http://dhss.delaware.gov/dph/files/organochlorpestfaq.pdf

61: https://www.downtoearth.org/articles/2009-03/68/sucralose-dangerous-sugar-substitute

62: https://www.endocrineweb.com/endocrinology/overview-thymus

63: http://www.bbc.co.uk/science/humanbody/body/factfiles/spleen/spleen.shtml

64: https://www.wsj.com/articles/heartland-food-products-to-buy-splenda-from-j-j-unit-1440529979

65: https://en.wikipedia.org/wiki/Neotame

66: http://sci-toys.com/ingredients/neotame.html

67: http://www.foodnavigator.com/Market-Trends/Neotame-wins-approval-in-Europe

68: http://www.ivyroses.com/Define/E954

69: http://www.ukfoodguide.net/e954.htm

70: https://www.ncbi.nlm.nih.gov/pmc/articles/PMC1469723/

71: https://www.ncbi.nlm.nih.gov/pubmed/3053447

72: https://pubchem.ncbi.nlm.nih.gov/compound/toluene#section=Top

73: http://www.sciencemag.org/news/1997/10/smoldering-battle-over-saccharin-heats

74: https://www.sciencemag.org/news/1997/11/saccharin-still-potentially-dangerous

75: https://www.sciencedaily.com/releases/2015/03/150317093142.htm

76: https://www.biology-innovation.co.uk/pages/human-biology/homeostasis/

77: https://www.sciencedaily.com/releases/2013/09/130922205933.htm

78: http://www.food-info.net/uk/e/e500.htm

79: http://www.ukfoodguide.net/e401.htm

80: https://en.wikipedia.org/wiki/Carbo-mer

81: http://www.food-info.net/uk/e/e524.htm

81: http://www.tandfonline.com/doi/abs/10.3109/10408449009089867

82: http://www.tandfonline.com/doi/abs/10.3109/10408449009089867

83: http://www.ivyroses.com/Define/E214

84: http://www.food-info.net/uk/e/e216.htm

85: https://pubchem.ncbi.nlm.nih.gov/compound/Butyl_4-hydroxybenzoate#section=Top

86: http://www.ivyroses.com/Define/E127

87: http://articles.mercola.com/herbal-oils/anise-oil.aspx

88: https://www.efsa.europa.eu/en/press/news/040929

89: https://en.wikipedia.org/wiki/Erythrosine

90: http://www.livestrong.com/article/460662-what-is-sodium-saccharin/

91: http://www.livestrong.com/article/22810-dangers-aspartame/

92: https://www.theatlantic.com/health/archive/2012/05/how-natural-is-stevia/257882/

93: http://www.bayneurope.com/e960-natural/

94: https://www.fda.gov/aboutfda/transparency/basics/ucm194320.htm

95: http://www.foodnavigator-usa.com/Suppliers2/More-companies-move-into-stevia-market

96: http://www.reuters.com/article/us-fda-stevia idUSN1841210720070918?feedType=RSS&feedName=healthNews

97: http://www.foodnavigator-usa.com/Regulation/FDA-tells-industry-whole-stevia-leaf-isn-t-GRAS-approved-food-additive

98: https://en.wikipedia.org/wiki/Rebaudioside_A

99: http://www.foodnavigator-usa.com/Regulation/Stevia-sweetener-gets-US-FDA-go-ahead

100: http://www.foodnavigator-usa.com/Suppliers2/Cargill-develops-flavor-solutions-for-stevia

101: http://www.foodnavigator-usa.com/Regulation/Steviol-glycosides-are-not-all-natural-says-new-class-action-lawsuit

102: http://www.foodnavigator.com/Market-Trends/Stevia-is-not-just-another-E-number-says-Euromonitor

**Primary Research**

http://ajcn.nutrition.org/content/88/6/1716S.full.pdf+html

http://link.springer.com/article/10.1007/s00217-015-2437-7

https://www.ncbi.nlm.nih.gov/pmc/articles/PMC4014048/

http://www.vladozlatos.com/project/files/pages/2218/8-.safety-of-sucralose.pdf

http://www.sciencedirect.com/science/article/pii/S0149763414002140

http://care.diabetesjournals.org/content/diacare/36/9/2530.full.pdf

https://www.ncbi.nlm.nih.gov/pmc/articles/PMC3853506/pdf/tjp0591-5727.pdf

http://www.mdpi.com/2072-6643/7/1/17/htm

http://care.diabetesjournals.org/content/diacare/36/12/e202.full.pdf

http://www.tandfonline.com/doi/pdf/10.1080/10937404.2013.842523?needAccess=true

https://www.hindawi.com/journals/jt/2013/372986/

https://www.nature.com/articles/srep09598

http://onlinelibrary.wiley.com/doi/10.1038/oby.2008.284/pdf

http://ajcn.nutrition.org/content/89/1/1.full.pdf+html

http://journals.plos.org/plosmedicine/article/file?id=10.1371/journal.pmed.1002195&type=printable

## Articles

https://www.ncbi.nlm.nih.gov/pmc/articles/PMC3185898/pdf/conc-18-213.pdf

https://www.organicconsumers.org/essays/gmo-food-antibiotic-laced-meat-and-high-fructose-corn-syrup-have-made-us-fattest-nation

http://www.theecologist.org/take_action/268653/sweet_truth_how_and_why_our_food_is_laced_with_sugar.html

http://www.mayoclinic.org/healthy-lifestyle/nutrition-and-healthy-eating/in-depth/artificial-sweeteners/art-20046936

http://www.independent.co.uk/life-style/health-and-families/health-news/sugar-free-diet-drinks-coke-not-aid-weight-loss-healthier-full-fat-research-study-a7507901.html

http://www3.imperial.ac.uk/newsandeventspggrp/imperialcollege/newssummary/news_3-1-2017-16-59-3

http://pediaa.com/difference-between-dextrin-and-maltodextrin/

http://content.time.com/time/health/article/0,8599,1931116,00.html

http://discovermagazine.com/2005/aug/chemistry-of-artificial-sweeteners

http://www.mintel.com/press-centre/food-and-drink/stevia-set-to-steal-intense-sweetener-market-share-by-2017-reports-mintel-and-leatherhead-food-research

http://www.scientificamerican.com/article/artificial-sweeteners-may-change-our-gut-bacteria-in-dangerous-ways/

http://www.checkdiabetes.org/glycogenesis/

https://www.efsa.europa.eu/en/topics/topic/sweeteners

https://authoritynutrition.com/sucralose-good-or-bad/

http://www.foodinsight.org/articles/everything-you-need-know-about-sucralose

https://www.infowars.com/neotame-13000-times-sweeter-than-sugar-and-more-toxic-than-aspartame/

https://www.scientificamerican.com/article/how-gut-bacteria-help-make-us-fat-and-thin/

http://www.nature.com/news/food-preservatives-linked-to-obesity-and-gut-disease-1.16984

http://www.nature.com/news/gut-brain-link-grabs-neuroscientists-1.16316

https://www.theguardian.com/business/2017/mar/27/brexit-sugar-beet-cane-tate-lyle-british-sugar

http://www.independent.co.uk/news/business/analysis-and-features/not-such-sweet-success-280263.html

http://articles.mercola.com/sites/articles/archive/2009/02/10/new-study-of-splenda-reveals-shocking-information-about-potential-harmful-effects.aspx

http://www.westonaprice.org/health-topics/dirty-secrets-of-the-food-processing-industry/

http://articles.mercola.com/sites/articles/archive/2012/03/28/neotame-more-toxic-than-aspartame.asp

http://www.bbc.co.uk/news/magazine-22758059

http://drhyman.com/blog/2013/09/26/fatty-liver-90-million-americans/

http://www.huffingtonpost.com/dr-mark-hyman/high-fructose-corn-syrup-dangers_b_861913.html

http://www.webmd.com/diet/features/your-hunger-hormones#1

https://www.agra-net.com/agra/foodnews/beverages/soft-drinks/eu-hfcs-production-to-increase-threefold-when-sugar-quotas-end-in-2017-217590.htm

https://en.wikipedia.org/wiki/Erythritol

https://en.wikipedia.org/wiki/Isomalt

https://en.wikipedia.org/wiki/Mannitol

https://en.wikipedia.org/wiki/Xylitol

https://en.wikipedia.org/wiki/Toluene

http://chemicalsareyourfriends.com/posts/synthetic-sweeteners-pt-2-sucralose-neotame-saccharin-and-special-natural-guest-stevia/

http://www.nature.com/news/sugar-substitutes-linked-to-obesity-1.15938

http://articles.mercola.com/sites/articles/archive/2008/12/16/stevia-the-holy-grail-of-sweeteners.aspx

https://www.theguardian.com/science/2013/feb/03/dopamine-the-unsexy-truth

https://www.theguardian.com/education/2016/sep/13/small-schools-turkey-twizzlers-underfunding-infant-free-school-meals

http://www.monbiot.com/2015/08/11/slim-chance/

https://www.theguardian.com/society/2014/jun/21/how-britain-got-so-fat-obese

http://www.nature.com/nature/journal/v486/n7403_supp/full/486S7a.htm

http://www.nature.com/nature/journal/v486/n7403_supp/full/486S2a.html

http://www.nature.com/news/2008/080326/full/news.2008.692.html

http://www.fao.org/ag/agn/jecfa-additives/specs/monograph10/additive-442-m10.pdf

https://www.sciencedaily.com/releases/2014/09/140917131634.htm

https://www.sciencedaily.com/releases/2016/07/160712130107.htm

https://www.sciencedaily.com/releases/2016/10/161024090351.htm

https://www.sciencedaily.com/releases/2013/05/130529190728.htm

https://www.britannica.com/print/article/270188

https://www.sciencedaily.com/releases/2008/02/080210183902.htm

 https://emergency.cdc.gov/agent/phosgene/basics/facts.asp

https://www.newscientist.com/article/mg13217960-400-shrunken-glands-spark-sweetener-controversy/

http://www.theecologist.org/investigations/health/268764/life_after_aspartame.html

https://www.theatlantic.com/magazine/archive/2017/01/the-sugar-wars/508751/

https://www.theatlantic.com/health/archive/2014/08/artificial-sweeteners-probably-okay/378937/

http://www.sciencemag.org/news/2014/09/artificial-sweeteners-may-contribute-diabetes-controversial-study-finds

http://www.worldhistory.biz/sundries/37289-food-additives-in-history.html

http://blog.euromonitor.com/2013/02/e960-stevia-may-be-an-additive-but-its-natural-sourcing-will-make-it-a-winner.html

http://articles.mercola.com/sites/articles/archive/2009/01/10/fda-approves-two-new-stevia-based-sweeteners.aspx

https://authoritynutrition.com/truvia-good-or-bad/

**Reports and reviews**

https://www.britishlivertrust.org.uk/liver-information/liver-conditions/non-alcohol-related-fatty-liver-disease/

http://www.thelancet.com/pdfs/journals/landia/PIIS2213-8587(15)00009-1.pdf

http://www.thelancet.com/pdfs/journals/lancet/PIIS0140-6736(14)61746-3.pdf

http://www.neotame.com/pdf/neotame_science_brochure_US.pdf

http://www.futuremarketinsights.com/reports/global-stevia-market

https://www.ncbi.nlm.nih.gov/pmc/articles/PMC3198517/

https://www.ncbi.nlm.nih.gov/pmc/articles/PMC2685866/

## Sustainability Websites

http://www.foodforlife.org.uk/

https://www.soilassociation.org/

## Corporate Websites

http://www.polyols-eu.com/home

https://www.givaudan.com/

## Other Websites

http://newsite.personalnutrition.org/WebSite/Home.aspx

http://www.sugar-and-sweetener-guide.com/e-number-index-for-sweeteners.html

# Chapter 8

## Sources

http://www.foodnavigator.com/Policy/Rosemary-extracts-get-final-EU-approval-for-food-preservation

http://www.organicherbtrading.com/getattachment/Products/ProductsPrice List/Price-list-page/Products/Rosemary/Rosemary-CO2-Extract-2016.pdf.aspx

https://www.nhrorganicoils.com/products.php?id=2855

http://www.telegraph.co.uk/news/earth/environment/11679681/Soil-Association-approved-use-of-unauthorised-pesticide-on-organic-crops.html

http://news.harvard.edu/gazette/story/2014/12/bacteria-churn-out-valuable-chemicals/

http://www.npr.org/sections/thesalt/2014/12/04/368001548/who-made-that-flavor-maybe-a-genetically-altered-microbe

https://pubchem.ncbi.nlm.nih.gov/compound/Calcium_dichloride#section=Top

http://www.food-info.net/uk/e/e509.htm

https://noshly.com/additive/e509/firming-agent-plus/509/#.WZ_ryD6QzIU

https://en.wikipedia.org/wiki/Calcium_chloride

https://www.cdc.gov/niosh/ipcsneng/neng1184.html

http://www.livestrong.com/article/299977-what-are-the-dangers-of-calcium-chloride-as-a-food-additive/

https://www.panna.org/sites/default/files/imported/files/PANmagSum09CocktailEffect.pdf

http://ec.europa.eu/environment/chemicals/effects/effects_en.htm

https://www.sciencedaily.com/releases/2011/06/110614131954.htm

## Crop Protection Association Website

http://www.cropprotection.org.uk/